Testimonials

"No matter the drama or crisis in your life, this book will open your eyes to the future and leave you 'Wide Awake'. Walk side by side with Mody as she moves forward on the path of life, using her experiences to share step by step strategies for rekindling your spirit and healing your soul."

John Forrest
Author - 10 editions, Chicken Soup for The Soul.

Wide Awake by Sara Mody is an honest, heartwarming and at times uproariously funny account of a woman who loses all yet gains in wisdom, self love and sheer chutzpah. A delightful, memorable read!!

Lissa M. Cowan

Sara is living proof that the experiences she shares in her book can help anyone in their lifelong journey as long as they are willing to open their own doors. This book will inspire and motivate readers to make positive changes in their lives no matter what challenges they face. Wide Awake is a testament to what is possible.

Vikram Vij

WIDE AWAKE

SARA MODY

Acknowledgements

Firstly, I would like to give a gigantic thank you to my family for their unwavering support and love and for believing in me. When I first mentioned writing a book to my father and mother, they both demonstrated confidence in me, and showed considerable patience through the writing process. Growing up, my parents taught me to stay focused and tackle obstacles so that I would accomplish anything I put my mind to. This book would not have been possible without my mother's editing skills and her love of literacy.

Mom, thank you for exposing me to the world of literacy and sharing your passion for reading with me. I have always admired you for constantly having a book or a crossword puzzle in your hand. My fondest childhood memory of you is when you religiously curled up in bed with me and read me stories. Your animated voices and passion for reading stories is a gift that I have learned and mastered from you and that I share with my students every day. When I read to my class I hear your voice. I share my passion for storytelling and the importance for learning to read with my students in hopes of sparking within their hearts that same passion for reading that I have. I dedicate this book to you as a way to express my gratitude for your dedication and focus in listening to me share my dream of creating this book and making it a reality. You are my favourite teacher and I aspire to be just like you.

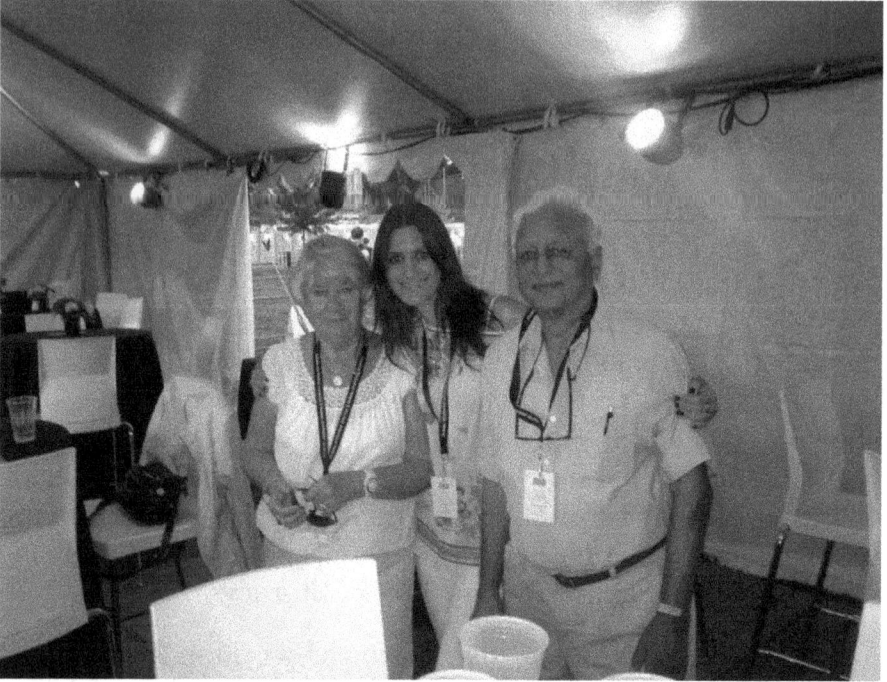

Mom and Dad

Dad, there are no words to describe how thankful I am for all you have given me. You are truly the man in my life that has been there supporting me and showing me how to be a better person. Daddy, you have been the saviour in my life fixing what falls apart and looking out for my best interests in every decision that I have made, whether good or bad. My fondest memory of you is the day you left your work to cheer me on at the end of my first cross-country race. Seeing your face at the finish line is a moment when I was proud to have you as my father and knew in my heart that you would always be there for me, loving me every step of the way, even when I doubt myself. You are my hero. Always. I hope I have made you proud.

Janaki, thank you for being my "rock" during all the difficult times that life has thrown my way. I admire your strength and determination and appreciate you always lending your ear when I need someone to listen, and for never judging me.

I want to acknowledge my dearest friend Natalie for her attentiveness in reading chapter after chapter of this book and giving me feedback. You have supported me from the beginning and have played a large part in this project with your suggestions and advice. You constantly listened and accepted my passion. I appreciate you sitting by my side in Starbucks and for assisting me with my technical difficulties while writing this book on my outdated laptop.

I give a big hug to Stephanie for listening, loving, and supporting me with my journey of self discovery. I cannot imagine my life without you by my side. You are like a sister to me. Thank you for always being there when I needed your help and hugs.

I owe so much to the success of publishing this book to John Forest. He is an author, a friend and my biggest mentor. John, I appreciate all of your advice while completing my book. Your thoughtful and frequent emails and words of wisdom gave me the strength and power to believe in myself. You gave me confidence when I had none. Thank you for sharing your expertise with me.

Thank you to my editor Lissa M. Cowan for your kind words and your flexibility with my project and vision. Your suggestions and professionalism shone through in every email I received from you. During the editing process I looked forward to receiving your words of wisdom on how to improve my writing and to make it the successful story it has now become.

Thank you to Lynn Simpson at Pine Lake Books for your patience and for helping me develop this book into a work of art that people can easily download and read. I very much appreciate your informative communications with me, and your great ideas and creativity.

I must also thank my counsellor Laura Elliot for providing me with a warm and comfortable space to heal. You are one of the most beautiful and genuine women that I have had the pleasure of sharing my whole story with in complete confidence. Thank you for your support, love, and words of encouragement. Being able to feel vulnerable and comfortable with you allowed me to come to terms with my situation and to move forwards. You have provided me with confidence and the ability to learn from my mistakes and become a stronger person. I owe you a case of bottled water.

A big thanks to Stephanie R., Amy T., Irina H., Cecila G., Liz O., Alex A., Tamara A., Jeff T., and Fouad M. Thank you to Matt Basile, Vikram Vij, Michael Smith, Joy McCarthy, Peter Neal, Mark McEwan and to every other Canadian chef that took time to autograph their cookbook for me and share their love of food with the world.

Thank you to all the amazing countries I visited, and for the experiences I brought home and cherish in my heart.

Thank you to the Canadian Breast Cancer Foundation, and to all my oncologists, surgeons and every medical doctor, nurse and hospital that has treated my cancer and provided the best health care possible to keep me living each day to the fullest.

Thank you to Starbucks for giving me a comfortable place to express myself and for providing me with warm cups of lattes and teas. Thank you to GoodLife Fitness for your amazing programs and instructors that encouraged me to find my passion in exercise and for inspiring me to stay healthy. A warm appreciation goes to Carol at Zawada Health for always providing me with hope and possibilities to attain a healthy and happy life through food options and lifestyle changes. You have saved my life twice and I am in total gratitude to you.

The connections and friendships that I developed along my journey have brought inspiration and hope into my life.

Thank you to all the wonderful people I have had the honour of meeting and who have touched my life in the simplest way. Whether or not you realize it, you have had a hand in shaping or creating a path for me to follow that has changed my life trajectory.

I am grateful for every individual that I meet, and everyone I will encounter in the future. Connections build new beginnings and create many destinies.

To everyone that has been affected by cancer, remember you are strong and beautiful. You can accomplish all that you desire if you put your mind, heart and soul into it. Think positively and fight to the end. Surround yourself with love and laughter.

Sara Mody

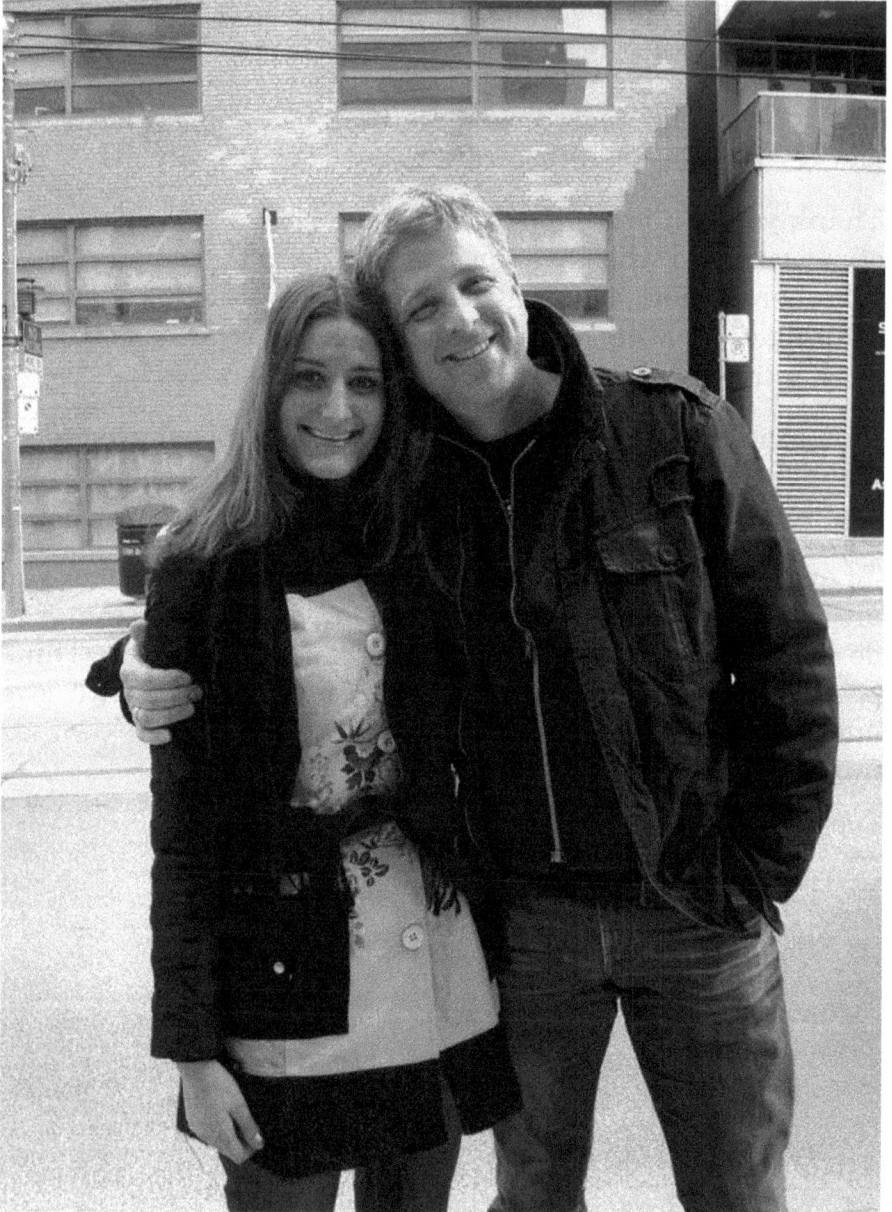

Peter Neal

Preface

I will never forget the moment my husband told me he no longer loved me. The man I trusted most in the world looked me in the eyes and calmly said that it was over.

Four years prior, when I made my vows, I trusted my husband with my life. At that time I knew that he loved and trusted me in exactly the same way. I never imagined those feelings could change for either of us. Divorce was something that happened to other people. Not us. Not me.

When I found out he was having an affair and our marriage was over, my entire being became submerged, as if I was underwater watching life happen above me. I could not fully make sense of what he said, and I could not bring myself to process the changes they implied. Suddenly, I understood what people meant when they talked about time standing still.

Two years prior, I had been diagnosed with breast cancer, and I thought nothing could top that in terms of emotional upheaval. I was wrong. When the reality of my failed marriage finally began to sink in, the emotional pain only grew worse. Every day I woke up to renewed pain. My thought process changed, pushing me through an endless cycle of ever-conflicting emotions. On top of this, I was not getting answers to any of the nagging questions I had. Eventually I began to blame myself for what was happening, convinced that had I done things differently, I could have prevented my marriage from failing. Before long I had stopped eating and sleeping, and as I lost my ability to think and function, I began to lose sight of myself.

Like separation, cancer had also changed me.

Although I was a vibrant, young woman, I suddenly had to make decisions that were literally a matter of life and death. Do I choose chemotherapy or radiation? Should I have a lumpectomy? These aren't things you think you'll have to decide at my age, yet I had no choice. I endured 30 rounds of radiation treatment and had a lumpectomy on my right breast. Days after my lumpectomy, I was already back in my classroom, and continued to work throughout my entire radiation treatment. Each day, after teaching my kindergarten students, I would drive 40 minutes to the hospital for my treatment and then drive myself back home at the end of the day exhausted.

Although this period of my life was incredibly difficult, the diagnoses forced me to take charge of my situation and immediately change my life. I bought a juicer, became a vegetarian, started doing yoga daily, and began to embrace every moment spent with my friends and family. I had a plan, a schedule, things to do, goals to accomplish, and a timeframe to follow. I felt strong and unstoppable.

When crisis strikes some people turn to sex, drugs, alcohol, and gambling to help them cope. Sure, it helps to alleviate the pain temporarily, but it does not make the pain go away. The pain is just compartmentalized into a box waiting to be revisited at a later time.

Although separation left me with the same desperate need for answers and healing as with cancer, there was no doctor to walk me through my pain and provide me with medication or a personalized step-by-step plan for recovery. Unlike my experience with cancer, I was given no prognosis, no pamphlets, and no timeline. I was in it alone. Even more than this was the knowledge that, unlike cancer, this was pain that had been inflicted on with me wilfully and knowingly by someone I loved and trusted.

Rather than focus on the damage the separation caused, I want to focus on the positives in my life. I'm certain that doing this helped me to heal faster. It took me four months before I started to notice that I was healing and experiencing happiness after my relationship had ended. Even this felt like a major accomplishment. Don't despair if it takes you longer. Everyone is different, and there is no deadline for recovery. I wish to stress however, that you have to take responsibility for yourself. In the end, it is up to you to set proactive goals that can lead you towards recovery.

During my separation I wanted desperately for a book that could guide me toward immediate relief. As the days went by, my lack of a strategy made me more and more anxious. I am a primary school teacher, not a counsellor, therapist, or a social worker. I do not have a degree in psychology and have no special training when it comes to mental and physical health; but I can honestly say that I made it through separation to a place of health and happiness. I believe that I am a survivor, not once but twice. As a teacher, I love telling stories. I read stories and teach children to create stories everyday in my job. Everyone has a story to tell and share and this is mine.

I hope that my experience will provide you with the support and encouragement you need to cope with whatever pain you're dealing with—be it emotional, physical, psychological or spiritual, and to heal your soul on a day-to-day and moment-to-moment basis. More than anything though, I hope you will feel less alone and less helpless as you read my account, and that you will find the strength to create your own unique plan and strategy—your own story for healing.

Chapter 1

Journal--Write! Write! Write!

"If your eyes are positive, you will like the world and if your tongue is positive, the world will love you."

-Author Unknown

My healing process began with a journal and a pen. I believe that writing by hand is an art form with advantages that typing on a computer doesn't offer. Writing in this way comes alive on paper, and provides a personal touch. Receiving a handwritten card or a letter in the mail is tangible, thoughtful, and brings you closer to the author or sender.

To begin to describe my journey, I think back to where most of my thoughts, inspirations, and healing first began. It was in a bookstore close to where I live that had become my place of peace. It was my quiet temple to reflect and meditate. It was where I researched to find answers on how to deal with the intensity of my pain. It was where I first discovered my idea for journaling. I remember being mesmerized by the colours, designs, and styles of different types of journals that were strategically placed at the checkout counter to be adopted and taken home.

One day, I was staring at the endless selection while sipping my Starbucks Chai Latte and trying to hear which journal called to me. It was the array of journals that made me realize I wanted to record and reflect my feelings onto paper. I wanted to convert my pain into words as though spilling directly from my body onto the page.

I brought the chosen journal home. I had no idea where to begin, yet knew I had to. That act of opening the journal to the first page was the step that got me journaling. Sentences started growing in length as my emotions poured onto the paper. Continuing to write and write, my mood began to change. I felt release and relaxation, and—for a time—my sadness lessened. This may sound crazy, yet I sensed that my journal was absorbing all of my sorrow. I trusted my journal, and I was beginning to appreciate and realize my thoughts as I wrote them. After completing my first entry, I leaned back on my couch and reread what I had written. Ironically, when I was writing, there was not a tear in my eye; however, rereading my thoughts as a whole brought tears to my eyes and made me realize just how much I needed to empty my heart's trauma and take the first step to recovery.

Over the ensuing weeks and months, my journal became my go-to girlfriend. As if I were confiding my deepest thoughts to a trustworthy friend who was not going to judge me or tell me I was crazy. Journaling was fast becoming a representation of my strength and allowing me to purge my pain. Slowly, I was developing a relationship with my journal. Concurrently, I was developing a new relationship with myself. I carried my journal everywhere with me. There was not a place I ventured, where my trusty journal was not within arm's reach, or should I say fingers' reach. I hugged it while on lunchroom duty at my school. Every night before I went to sleep, I placed it at my bedside. Sometimes, I even put it in my gym bag in case I needed to write down any unexpected emotions. I became extremely reliant on this traditional way of writing to deal with trauma. Whenever I felt alone, unhappy, confused, or downright miserable, my journal was there for me to quickly refocus my thoughts in an organized and therapeutic manner.

In time the journal took on different forms as I brought it with me to different locations. I began recording positive quotes I had heard or read, and glued into it pictures or emails from loved ones that made me smile or gave me hope when I was crumbling. To help me through the process, I started writing down websites, books, movies, speakers, and workshops that were recommended to me by friends and colleagues. On the very last page on the bottom line, I wrote down the present date and recorded one thing I was grateful for until I worked myself up to the top of the page. Then when that page was full, I went to the next page. As days turned into weeks, and weeks turned into months, I noticed how grateful and appreciative I was for so many things in my life. If I yearned for an instant smile and reminder of the many wonderful experiences, and people that surrounded me, then I would just look at my list.

Little did I know that the most valuable and astonishing healing was just around the corner.

As I continued to write, I was unaware that I was creating a document of the person I was becoming. As the months went on and my pages filled with words and snippets of me, I was building my own awareness of my positive progress. I remember one day in particular, curled up in my bed with my cat and my journal, I hit "writer's block." I suddenly felt as though I was a broken record and that I had said everything that needed saying. I stared at my journal and wracked through my brain for something to put down on the paper. Yet the more I concentrated on finding a thought, an idea or an emotion, the more I just kept drawing blanks. I decided to read my whole journal from beginning to end. There was a part of me that was scared to see the words describing my hurt and relive those moments, yet I was curious enough to give it a go. As I began rereading my words, I admit to feeling nostalgic as memories of my distress filled me all over again. As I continued reading, it became apparent that my pain was less intense and I was becoming stronger. My journey was a viewpoint to my evolution, healing, and rediscovery of who I was.

Psychotherapist Maud Purcell wrote an article on the benefits of journaling where she mentions that journaling has "a positive impact on our physical well being." She explains that writing activates the left hemisphere of the brain, the rational half. Furthermore, while your left side is occupied, you are allowing your creative side to come alive and activate your imagination. As a result, the mental stresses of the day will take a back seat as you explore your being and the world around you.

Writing is a powerful exercise that helps transform thoughts and emotions into words on a page. When you reread your words, it feels as though you are thinking, searching, connecting, and discovering deep realizations about yourself and of reality. Reading words that you have written about yourself is an extremely powerful process.

When I reread my journal, I noted that what I was doing was reading positive statements that I wrote to myself to help me heal. I was convincing myself to heal and rise above the pain. These simple positive sentences made me smile. Words are powerful and contagious! Here are some examples of what I wrote to myself.

> Be Positive Sara ... Move On. ... You deserve better ....
> Are you happy Sara?
>
> Forget the past... Forgive yourself... I love myself ... I am my own person.
>
> I am joyous and happy ... I approve of myself exactly as I am ....
>
> Trust your gut... Heal yourself... Spoil yourself... Laugh...

> Trust in the power of destiny and time... You will survive... You are strong.

Rereading this list that I wrote a month after my spouse left, made me realize that I was strong. I must have been strong to write such positive and powerful affirmations one month after separation. A quote by Anna Freud reads, "I was always looking outside myself for strength and confidence, but it comes from within. It is there all the time." I now feel that deeply in my bones.

Time and time again, I suggested to my friends who were also walking the road of separation to buy a journal. It was the one piece of advice that I shared over and over again. A journal is affordable, accessible, and good for any age, gender, and race. It is portable, and easy and has long-term results. If there is no other advice in this book that speaks to you, try journaling. You will not regret it.

I noticed when reflecting on my journal that I had added events from my marriage that made me unhappy or had raised red flags that I had ignored. As time passed and the more I reflected on my situation, the more I began to heal, and I realized that I had not been happy in my marriage. At the same time, I had friends and family reminding me of situations that occurred or things I had said to them that I had forgotten while involved in my marriage because I simply chose to forget or ignore. As I started writing down my feelings, I slowly walked down memory lane and began recalling events that indicated I was not in a healthy committed marriage. It was not the type of marriage that I wanted or deserved, yet only after it was over and I had begun to heal, could I admit that to myself.

One thing that I feel connects to journaling in a big way, and something I also did to heal, was meditation. After my separation I started researching this ancient exercise and then practising it. I say *exercise* because I see it as an emotional and spiritual workout for the soul and the mind. Yes, we have a brain, which is an organ made up of matter, yet the mind cannot be touched or seen. It is the mind, not the brain that requires emptying, exploring, detoxing, and stretching. Meditation allows for this release and promotes healing.

Amy, a high school friend gave me a fantastic book to read called *Heal Your Mind, Rewire Your Brain* by Patt Lind-Kyle. This book enlightened and delighted me as I flipped through its endless pages. The book mentions topics such as meditation, the difference between the mind and the brain, Buddhism, and The Enneagram. In her book, she makes an amazing statement about the difference between the mind and brain: "The mind is what the brain does." She believes that it is the mind alone that elicits healing and changes in our body. Therefore, it is meditation that exercises our mind.

I see journaling as a form of meditation. You are not sitting in a cross-legged position with the lights off, eyes closed, yet you are encouraging the healthy flow of thoughts, whether positive or negative to be emptied from your mind. Lind-Kyle writes that intention, attention, receptivity, and awareness are the four fundamentals to training your mind and balancing your mental and emotional being. These fundamentals can also be applied to journaling.

Intention

When you journal, you have an *intention* in mind. You are making a conscious effort to hold a pen in your hand and write.

Attention

Attention is what you give when you type or write words from your mind onto a tangible space. You are focused on your goal or project. It has purpose.

Receptivity

This allows each of you to perceive the thoughts that float around your mind. You accept, encourage, and allow these thoughts to occur and to flow onto the paper. You recognize their being and give them relevance by recording them. You are validating their existence.

It is important to open your mind to all thoughts that you have, whether positive or negative. Even if it means writing words onto the paper and crying or if it stirs up feelings of depression, loss, anxiety, or pain, you must tolerate and give residence to every thought in your mind. It is there for a reason, and, like a caged animal, it wants to escape. So, trust yourself and believe you are strong and take a chance and open that cage and release it.

Awareness

This is where you begin to become aware of what you have written and are feeling. At the same time, you are becoming aware of people around you whether negatively or positively. It is the one tool that I found to be the most interesting when journaling and emptying out my mind. It is now that you must be attentive and observe that you have inner thoughts and emotions, and while it is critical to accept and experience them, it is also equally important to keep them "at bay." Emotions will gush like an erupting volcano and being aware of this explosion is key; however, it is critical not to get carried away with your thoughts and possibly displaying some erratic behaviour that could have negative consequences.

Journaling is the key to self-reflective healing, building self esteem, and reducing stress. By this time you might be asking yourself, "How do I journal?" When I was trying to think of a way to help people journal, I myself did not know where to start, so I would just tell someone to begin writing and the rest will follow. However, being an elementary school teacher, I am also passionate about teaching others and providing the tools and strategies to help foster success, so I began researching websites to see if I could find some helpful tips about journaling.

I found a wonderful website called, *The Tiny Buddha* that suggests writing about where you are right now in your present moment. I agree with this completely. Your journal is nothing more than a record or document of your present state of being. You are longing to get those negative feelings and dump them out of your system. Another valid point from this website is to record your thoughts as they form in your mind without making yourself aware of what you are writing. I have discovered that this allows any bias to filter free expression of my emotions and thoughts. You are not writing for a newspaper, so there is no reason to worry or stress yourself out about being a perfectionist. Your thoughts come alive as your write them in your journal. Remember that you are writing in the moment, experiencing the moment, and accepting all that you are, mistakes and all!

I had the opportunity to see Deepak Chopra at Roy Thompson Hall in Toronto deliver a seminar titled, *The Future of Well Being*. One of his theories was about "self reflection" and he spoke about the importance of *self-reflecting* or self-awareness. He said the more we reflect on choices, thoughts, feelings, and beliefs, the more we become the observer of our present situation. We begin to see reality and questions are answered. Deepak believes that the process of "reality making" is a positive process, or as I like to put it, a *healing journey*. You make the choice to reshape the way your brain thinks, and your state of being. Pretty cool, eh!?

My personal favourite is to build a collection of positive quotes or messages that make you smile. *The Tiny Buddha* refers to it as cultivating an attitude of gratitude. I kept my gratitude separate from the rest of the thoughts in my journal. I began recording the date daily at the back of my journal and worked backwards, starting from the bottom line towards the top. Whether deep or simple, each day I wrote down things I was grateful for. For example, I was grateful for my family, friends, health, career, and home. While at the same time, I was also grateful for chocolate, bumblebees, trees, shampoo, my cats' purrs, my bracelets, or having no allergies. I wrote down anything that made me smile. If it made me smile, then I was grateful for it. I continued to record song titles I had heard that brought me happiness, or words, websites, books, cards, and emails that I printed off and literally glued into my journal that brought contentment to my world. ANYTHING!

Just remember that there is no limit to what you can write down and no right or wrong answer. It's wonderful to know that whenever you sense a moment of weakness, you can open your journal and remind yourself of all the things you have to be grateful for. You will see that your list will grow daily. Record anything that brings happiness to your life and has meaning to you. The first thing I did was glue a photo of my parents in the front of my journal. They were the most important people in my life and brought me all the love and support I needed during my process of healing.

In addition to all of these wonderful benefits, keeping a journal allows you to track patterns, trends, improvements, and growth over time. When current circumstances appear insurmountable, you can look back on previous dilemmas that you have since resolved. It's important to stay honest with yourself when you write or read your thoughts. Stay true to yourself and record everything you are experiencing and feeling. Facing the truth is difficult, but is necessary if you want to heal. Journaling is a healthy alternative to getting rid of the mental tensions that you have accumulated. Think of it as your mind's way of releasing. Journaling allows you the opportunity to develop self-awareness: The key to moving forward to a positive new beginning.

Recap

- Give yourself a pat on the back for choosing this book and telling yourself, YES you are going to get through the hurt, betrayal, frustration, and confusion. Make an effort to heal yourself naturally and take your life back.

- If you are sitting alone and having those urges to cry and drown your sorrows. STOP. Get out of the house, breathe the fresh air, buy your favourite comfort food or beverage and make a trip to the nearest bookstore. Treat yourself to a new journal and a funky pen and begin the journey of self-awareness, reflection, and healing.

- Collect pictures, photographs, quotes, websites, and anything that you think will put a smile on your face. Start to record these moments in your journal.

- Think of one thing you are grateful for today and WRITE IT DOWN! Remember to do this every day. Be creative and have fun.

- Think of places that give you peace or inspire you to write and be alone with your thoughts. Perhaps check out a local café or nearby library to see if you could make that space your own. Make time for you, to write and reflect.

NOW you are on your way to taking control of your happiness and moving on to a new and improved life. I am proud of you. You should be too!!

Chapter 2

Family and Friends

"Cherish your human connections - your relationships with friends and family."

-Barbara Bush

The actor Michael J. Fox once said, "Family is not an important thing. It's everything."

Well, that pretty much sums up how I feel about my family, and also my friends.

Parents:

I can not overstate the role that my parents had in helping me heal. My parents were my backbone, my anchor, and my escape from a harsh reality. Throughout my healing I was on the phone with my mother and father constantly. I desperately needed their support and so kept reaching out. Every time I called, they reassured me that I would be all right and that this was for the best. I depended on their words of encouragement, praise, and hope. They did not let me down.

Home:

During this time, one place I would escape to was my parents' home. I grew up in a small city north of Toronto called Orillia. Because I had spent my childhood and adolescence in this small town and had experienced many positive, and happy moments there, it was comforting for me to go back.

To assuage the pain I would sit on my parents' deck and reflect on my childhood memories.

As a child, I participated in ballet classes, summer and music camps, drum lessons, baking classes, and tennis lessons. By the time, I finished high school, I had a lifeguarding license, part-time jobs, and I was serious about ballet, and modelling. This foundation and exposure to all kinds of extracurricular activities, gave me a taste for other countries and cultures. By the time I graduated high school, I had already travelled to India, Holland, Scotland, Florida, Belgium, Portugal, and had visited many historical monuments. I saw and was in awe of the Taj Mahal, and witnessed the story of one girl's struggle and strong sense of self through journaling when I visited Anne Frank's house.

My parents saw me perform in school musicals, watched me run in cross country races, attended synchronized swimming events, and basically never missed a single event I participated in. My mother would remind me of how she worked at the bingo hall to send me to Bermuda with my high-school band. My parents were there when I changed careers. They held my hand when I was diagnosed with breast cancer in 2009. Now during my separation, it was my parents endless supply of love and support that I depended on to refuel my emotions.

Going back to my childhood and surrendering myself to my parents' supportive and unconditional love reminded me that I was in a place of love and that I was safe. During the first few months following the breakup I spent many hours on their deck, soaking in the warm sun, and listening to the symphony of birds cracking sunflower seeds with their beaks. My parents' backyard was a place of solitude and stillness for my thoughts. It was a place to reflect and be at peace with my thoughts. Being surrounded by nature reminded me of my connection to nature, which started when I was a child, and of how grateful I was to be alive and to witness such beauty.

In that garden I remembered that my childhood was spent building forts from recycled wood, wire, and any other garbage I could get my hands on, while my mother reminded me of the stray animals I used to bring home to nurture with the hope of keeping them as a pet.

Revisiting my parents' home and backyard reminded me of the person I was. It reminded me of the kind, strong, and loving person that I am.

I know it was difficult for them to share my depression, especially when they too were experiencing loss, anger, and betrayal. It is astonishing how much pain and sacrifice a family will endure for those they love. Families can provide unconditional love and endless support. My family definitely provided me with that and much more. My mother and father were my strength and my hope.

If you have that kind of relationship with your family, then it is crucial to seek out help from them. Do not be ashamed to ask for help! Also, I want to stress that family does not imply that they must be blood relations. Over the years, the definition of what a family consists of has evolved. Our social conventions, values, lifestyles, and tolerances have strengthened, evolved and, for the most part have been accepted. I am reminded of this everyday when I teach my students to accept and understand differences. As an educator who teaches children to love and accept everyone, I cherish and uphold these values. Please remember that receiving unconditional love from family, regardless of what that family might consist of, makes the process of healing stronger.

I have so many people in my extended family that have helped me on my healing path. The following is a list of those who were there the most when I needed them, and of what they stood for at the time, and still do today.

Janaki: Strength

My sister had a strong hand in helping me to recover by supporting me at my time of need. She is the "grab life by the balls" kind of gal, and so it wasn't surprising to me that she was on the phone to me immediately, encouraging, and supporting me with her strength.

It was her impulsiveness and spontaneity that led us to take off for the Christmas holiday to Costa Rica. She convinced me that I needed a vacation and to get away from the situation and be with family, and with her. I remember thinking that perhaps a trip was not the best thing for me. I was constantly crying, not eating, depressed, and angry at the world. Who in their right mind would want to travel with me? Only a loving sibling would!

It is my sister's unconditional love for me that shone through on that trip. The last thing I wanted was to ruin her vacation and experiences in Costa Rica due to my negative and depressed demeanor. Yet every time I woke up at four in the morning crying my eyes out or went to the pool to meditate, she made me feel as though it was okay. I must admit that I was not the best "all inclusive" travelling companion at the resort as I barely ate and was too afraid to drink in case it caused more depression. Yet, she listened to my every word and was patient, which gave me hope. She never once made me feel like a burden or that my questions were redundant. Janaki might have felt it, but she never once elicited an emotion of impatience to me, not even once!

She wanted so much for me to enjoy myself and to make it a memorable experience for me that she chose an activity that she knew was outside my comfort level. After she kept pushing at me to experience ATV-ing. It was the first time since my sadness took control that I smiled, laughed, and felt free. The adrenalin that raced through my spirit was like nothing I had felt before. As we sped through mud, past trees, rocks, fields, and over concrete, I remember staring at my sister's back and saying to myself:

"Thank you Janaki for believing and supporting me. I am so grateful to have a sister like you, who not only picked me up when I was down, but who helped me go the extra mile in my process of healing. "

I encourage you to seek out your own "Janaki", whoever that might be and find comfort and strength in their words.

Friends:

As I've said many times before, my family helped me heal in so many ways, yet I should also mention the importance of loyal friends, who, I consider family.

According to Dictionary.com, a friend is "a person attached to another by feelings of affection or a person that gives support or assistance." Who are your friends? This is an ongoing process. People change. Our values change, our experiences broaden, our knowledge grows, our expectations are created and our visions begin to predict the lives we want to live and with whom we want to live it. Choosing good friends and knowing who your friends are is one of the most important but most difficult processes in life. Like families, friendships are key relationships that help us through life. What makes a friendship so important is having a relationship with someone who has your best interests at heart and loves you for you, as hopefully, a family member would. I am not talking about acquaintances or fair weather friends. I'm talking about a friend who is there for you during the good and the bad times and wants nothing more for you than to be happy and healthy.

My truest friends, the ones I hold dearest and would travel to the ends of the earth with, are friends who have been there through my worst times. They are the friends that have proven themselves to me and love me for me. They are the friends that aren't just in my life when the times are good, happy, and fun, but rather, those that have held my hand, dried my tears, listened to my despair, given me hope and most importantly, been there in mind, spirit and soul, even when they were probably wishing they were somewhere else.

It took me to the age of 37 to learn about what I like to call "Friendship Spring Cleaning." I had to filter out those that felt that I was too draining to deal with during my separation. True friends will never make you feel bad about what you are going through or make you feel that you are an inconvenience in their life, but rather they will encourage you to call them and inform you constantly that they are there for you, and will go to extreme lengths to support you and love you, even though they might not understand your feelings.

To give you a short history about why friendships are so critical to me, I'd like to share a story with you. Growing up I found it difficult to build good friendships with girls. It wasn't that I wasn't a good friend, but rather, I was too gullible and forgiving. I used to have friends who took advantage of me and made me feel used. I never felt as though anyone missed me or wanted to spend time with ME! I was constantly doing and saying anything in order to have others accept me and care for me. Yet, at the time I did not love myself and I was drawing people close to me that didn't have my best interests at heart. It was not until later in life that I realized what it felt like to be taken advantage of, and be discarded so quickly by those that I thought were my closest friends. It was not until the tables had turned and there were days that I needed a favour, forgiveness, support or love that the feelings were not returned.

Friendship has no time limit. It does not matter if you went to kindergarten with someone and grew up with them, or you have only known them a couple of months. A real friend is someone that sticks by you and will go to great extremes to ensure you are happy and cared for. Quite simply put, they have your best interests at heart. It is the hardships and tragedies in life that expose your friends for who they really are.

The Benefits of Friendship

There is much research out there about how quality friendships promote happiness. Surrounding yourself with positive and loving friends will create happiness and slowly take over that emptiness you may feel in your heart after a breakup or other difficult life transition. A recent study by Harvard University shows that breast cancer patients with no friendship networks are four times more likely to die from the disease than those with ten or more close friends.

When I was diagnosed with breast cancer, my doctor suggested that I join a support group to help me cope with the changes brought by cancer. I was given materials that outlined how support groups helped patients reduce their depression and stress and improve self-worth.

It is interesting when I think back to the advice that was offered to me about joining a support group, and how easy it was for me to say I didn't want to join such a group. In my heart, I felt that I did not need a support group because of all the loving family and friends in my life. I felt that I had my own support group to help me deal with my issues and cope.

Signs of a Good Friend

Constantly moving in and out of your life, friends are a revolving door. There are those who make an impression for the short time they are with you, and those who—no matter what—are in it for the long haul. Every friend that we have in our lives serves a purpose, offering us life lessons that we can grow from. As our lives evolve and our values, opinions, and beliefs shift, so do our expectations of friendships and our definition of the word *friend*. I firmly believe that a good friend always loves you for who you are, and will always put your needs before their own. It is the little actions friends take that can demonstrate how much they care about you.

Separation led me to this epiphany on the importance of friendship, and so it is my hope that whatever losses or pain you are going through—that you will promise to surround yourself with people who care about you, love you, and who *have your back*!

Good friends will also encourage you to make positive changes in your life to help you heal. Positive people surrounded me, helping me open up without feeling judged. My true friends listened to me, offering supportive advice. A few months after my breakup, I was also bonding with friends who had or were experiencing the loss of a marriage in their own life, and who understood and accepted my pain. It was comforting to hear them as they shared advice and support. Releasing all my insecurities, emotions, thoughts, and anxieties to these dear ones reminded me that I was not alone. They gave me hope as they assured and promised me that I would heal and move on. Having good friends gave me answers to my questions and allowed me to make sense of what had happened. They were helping me face my shaken, yet beautiful life—wounds and all.

My idea of a friend

Friends are people who are...

- Loyal and without hesitation will pick me up when things get tough even at their own expense.
- Supportive through my good and bad times.
- Not judgmental and accepting (including my faults).
- Kind towards me and demonstrates respect towards me.
- Constantly showing me that they enjoy spending time with me because they want to be with me.
- Honest and willing to call a *spade a spade*, even though the truth hurts.
- Accepting of me and encourages me to always be myself.
- Loving towards me and makes me smile and laugh.
- Wonderful beings that I am addicted to spending time with because of how they make me feel.

During my marriage, I had many wonderful friends. Party friends, low-key friends, work friends, high school friends, and many acquaintances from different backgrounds. I had many girlfriends with whom to explore all that Toronto—a bustling, cultural metropolis—had to offer a young woman. I was what you might consider a *social butterfly,* and rarely if ever did I turn down the opportunity to try something new with a girl pal of mine. Yet, when things got really ugly for me, there were some friends who let me down.

To be fair I understand that not everyone is able, or knows how to offer exactly what is needed in terms of support. That's why it's important to decide exactly what you need from your friends by telling them how they can help you heal. I drew my own conclusions about whom my friends were based on who was willing to go the distance compared to those that were not.

At the same time as I was discovering what friends were or were not *there* for me, something magical happened that I hadn't expected. I was making friends along the way that would later become influential in my life.

Stephanie - Love

Words cannot express or ever be enough to describe my gratitude to one of the most astonishing woman I have ever met. I met her one summer at an Annual General Meeting for teachers in downtown Toronto in which we were both elected delegates. She sat in front me, crocheting an endless amount of different creative projects, such as, coasters, cat toys, scarves, and blankets. I asked her to show me how crocheting worked and with her kind heart and patient soul, she began to teach me the art of crocheting. I learned that she was also engaged, and was planning her wedding. Back then I was still married and was able to share my own stories of how I planned my wedding. As it turned out her partner and my partner shared common names. Yet that's not all we had in common. Turns out, her wedding was not to be and, looking back, it seemed like a sign of things to come for me.

As we became close friends, and she confided in me, I learned that her fiancé was unfaithful to her months before her BIG day, and her wedding was now off. Watching this gorgeous bride-to-be have her heart broken and dreams shattered beneath her broke my heart too. I tried to be there for her as best as I knew how. Having never had to deal with such a heavy blow, I did not have the authentic experience and knowledge to share with her on how to deal with her pain. All I knew was that I loved her and was there for her. As the months passed, she became stronger and our friendship blossomed. Of course, we were unaware at the time that I would experience the same ordeal with my own marriage. My husband would be unfaithful and my marriage would end.

So, when things did fall apart for me, it was Stephanie, having been through the process, who became my lighthouse in the fog. She was the one I called at the early hours of the night as I sobbed on my pillow. She was my anchor in a world of nonsense and denial. Stephanie shared tools, support, and advice to help me heal. She answered my questions and reached out to me every day. Always providing me with love and acceptance, this incredible woman even helped me predict events that were yet to come, sharing her experience and her stories with me. She would always go out dancing with me and meet me for dinner at Pizza Rustica, my favourite pizza place where I would drown my sorrows with cheese, wine, and chocolate dessert before dancing my bottom off. Stephanie was always there, offering me a place to stay, a book to read, a quote, time, patient advice, as she told me I was strong and I would get through it.

I'll never forget Stephanie's response when I asked her what she considered her most influential strategies or survival tactics.

If I'm truly honest with myself," she said, hesitating, "I would have to say it was when I looked at my situation for what was truly occurring. Facing reality and accepting its existence helped me to finally move forward. Feeling appreciation for what was real NOW in my life. Feeling grateful for my friends, my house, my job, my health.... So many things to be grateful for. I also reminded myself that there was *better* out there for me. This idea empowered me and gave me strength.

Stephanie taught me that people come into our lives for a reason. She made a statement to me one day that blew my mind and made me understand the true meaning of friendship. It was such a sincere comment, so selfless. She said, "I believe that I went through my breakup to help you go through yours."

Stephanie, thank you for comforting, counselling, guiding, and loving me every day through my separation. Thank you for picking up the phone in the morning, the afternoon or in the middle of the night to listen to me crying, and helping me to sleep again. Your patience and support was overwhelming and you never gave up on me. You never told me that I was emotionally draining or made me feel that I was a nuisance. Stephanie you are truly a friend and I am so grateful to have you in my life.

Cecila – Loyalty

Cecila was the wife of my ex-husband's best friend who also worked at the fire department. Let me clarify something about my relationship with Cecila. I knew of her and had met her a few times, yet I really didn't *know* her as a friend. It was not until her marriage fell apart months before mine that I reached out to this smart, beautiful woman. How it started was that one day I messaged her on Facebook to tell her I was there for her and not to hesitate to ask me for help. A month later, I was also going through the same thing and we were mirroring each other's feelings, of fear and confusion. Needless to say we bonded immediately. We compared marriage stories and began gathering and helping each other put the pieces of our scrambled lives together. We would share common themes and help each other come to a conclusion about what was true or untrue. Together we felt betrayed and deceived by our husbands, and together we helped each other make sense and provided comfort.

Every week we would call each other and listen to each other's stories, offering the other a shoulder to lean on. Even though she was going through the same thing, she was there for me, in a totally present and loving manner. She listened to me as a friend that could sympathize with my pain. We leaned on and empowered each other.

Irina -- Honesty

I used to see Irina in my Kombat class at Goodlife. She worked out in front of me and always had a smile on her face and a good word to say to those around her. Her bubbliness and confidence drew me to her. I began talking to her when I went to the gym, and through our ramblings discovered that we were almost neighbours, and both enjoyed similar social interests: dancing, movies, and my personal favourite—comedy clubs. One day I bumped into her at my bookstore and we exchanged numbers, making a plan to go for dinner and to a comedy show.

A year later, during my separation Irina constantly checked up on me and suggested that we take a trip together to Spain. She told me that I deserved a trip and a chance to get away. We spent ten days together and bonded as if we had known each other for years. During this time she was my crutch, my strength, and my reason for being. Irina promised me to tell me "like it was" and not to sugar coat anything. I utterly respected and adored her for her honesty.

After days of ordering and drinking pitchers of sangria and eating tapas, shopping in Madrid, and then dancing until six in the morning, she and I decided to chill in our rented flat in Barcelona located on La Rambla. I remember this as though it was yesterday. Overtired and high on the sights and sounds of the past day, I checked my email to see if my father had sent me any paper work on my separation. For a while I had been waiting for the document, related to the possession of my house, to be signed. Low and behold there was something. I was so nervous that I asked Irena to look and tell me what was on it. For months I had been waiting for my then-husband to sign the paperwork that would finalize our separation, yet at that moment I as too afraid to even look. I paced back and forth, my heart racing and my palms sweating like crazy.

She scrolled to the bottom on the page. Looking up at me with a wide smile on her face, she said, "He signed it."

I broke down with tears of joy and relief, and I could feel my body lifting as though from my chest. She was also crying as she gave me the best heartfelt hug I've ever received.

As she hugged me, she kept repeating, "The house is yours. He signed the papers. You are free Sara. You are free."

She suggested we go out that afternoon and celebrate with drinks and tapas. What a friend! She had dedicated hours of her time listening to me ramble on about my marriage and about signs that I had seen but chosen to ignore. We laughed, clinked glasses, ate delicious tapas, and bonded even more. What a celebration! Once again we strolled home around six in the morning! Thank you Irina for always seeing the good in me and for making me feel as though I matter. You are constantly opening up to me, and I am grateful everyday for your presence in my life.

Amy -- Thoughtfulness

Amy is the friend with whom I have shared the most memories. Outgoing, loving, open, and loyal, she and I would perform in high-school talent shows, go to school dances, work on school projects, and spend many weekends bonding and laughing. We stayed in touch over the years and she has always been one of my favourite childhood friends. Her relationship also ended when she discovered that her partner was unfaithful to her. Since Amy had already been through a break up and was one of my closest friends, it was not surprising that she was another confidante during my emotional ride.

One time I remember her inviting me to go to the movies with her and her friends, or to come over to watch movies at her place. Her attempts of inclusiveness always made me feel loved, comfortable, and needed. My most favourite memory of Amy showing her love, patience, and support towards me was when she gave me a makeover in her bathroom.

"Sara, this is the best thing that could happen to you, and months from now you'll see why," she said as she applied mascara to my lashes.

Amy showed me that I was beautiful, strong, and a survivor. She promised me that things happened for a reason and they did!

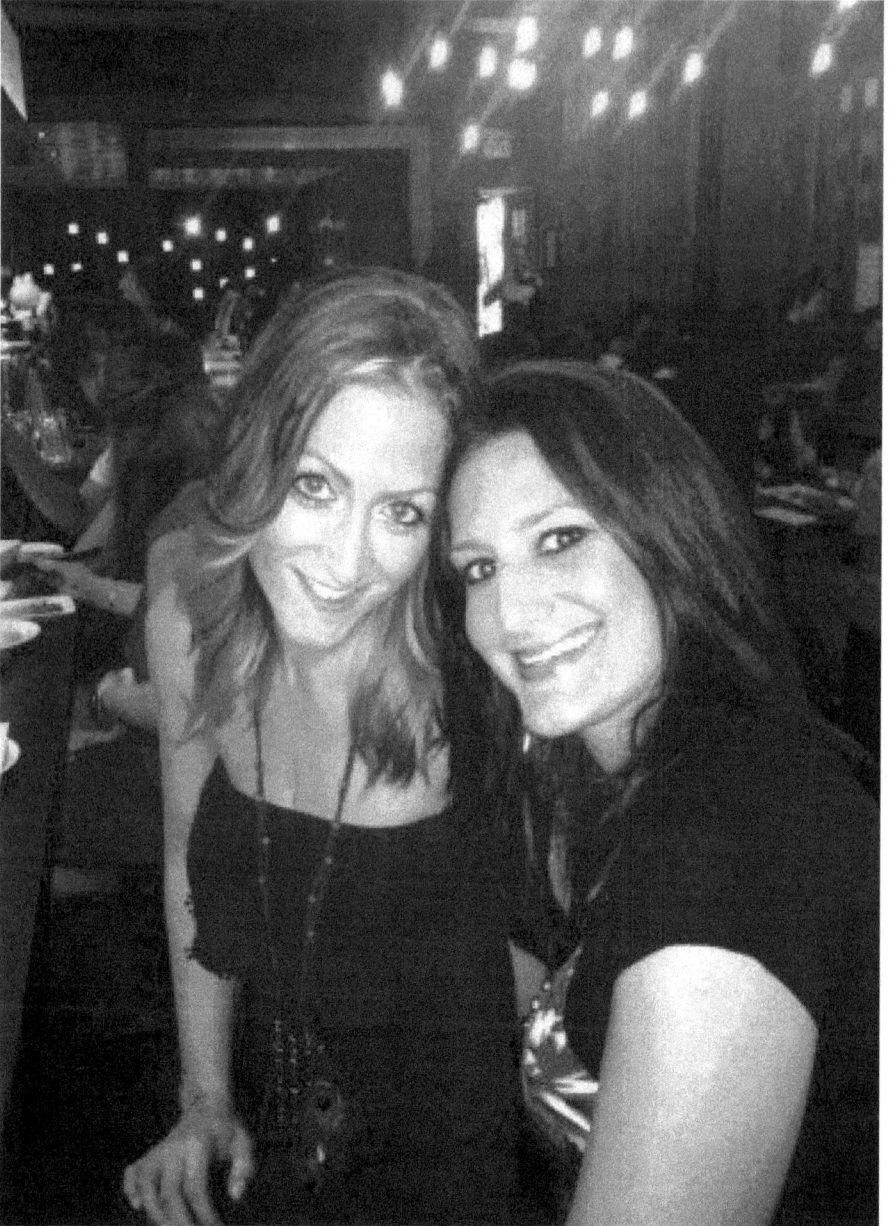

Amy and I discovering new restaurants

Liz -- Positivity

I met Liz on St. Patrick's Day—a perfect time to meet an energetic, fun-loving Irish woman. I was with a date and we were celebrating the occasion with pints of Guinness, kilts, pub grub, and Celtic music. Coming out of the washroom, or should I say stumbling out of the washroom with a big happy smile on my face, I literally fell onto this gorgeous woman who caught me before I landed on the floor. Her positive energy was infectious and that gave me the courage to not only thank her for catching me and preventing me from hurting myself, but it caused me to open up to her about my separation. She immediately complimented me, supported me, and made me feel that life was going to turn out all right for me. Turns out she had been with someone for many years, and confided in me that she had recovered too and eventually felt herself again. I knew I was meant to meet her that night.

The first time we went out was to an event at a museum. We talked all night long and exchanged dating stories and laughed the night away, not realizing that hours had passed. I knew from that night on that we would be good friends. Today Liz is one my closest and loyal friends. She always looks out for me and takes care of me. Confident and positive in nature, she draws so many to her. I have met a slew of people through Liz and would fly to the moon for her.

So many amazing women have inspired me to stay strong and have showed me through their actions that they loved me and assured me that I was better off and deserved better. And so here are some more I'd like to recognize:

Thank you Angela for your cups of tea, your hugs, and for helping me to learn about loving myself all over again.

Thank you Jenn for bringing me leftovers to work and for your loving, spontaneous texts to let me know that you thought of me, and that my happiness mattered to you.

Thank you Brenda for allowing me to enter your classroom every morning as you listened to my endless updates, and for sharing your strength and never giving up on me.

Natalie, I want to thank you for always being available in the mornings at work, and when I needed a friend to listen to my problems and help me eat carrot cake at our cafe.

As you can see, many friends have contributed to healing through my difficult times, and have loved me in many different ways. It is important to see that (even though) they all showed their support in many diverse ways, the most important common trait they all shared is that they never gave up on me!

Please remember to be grateful for the relationships you have and will make along the way. Every relationship offers something valuable to you and people come into your life for a reason. When in the depths of heartache it is critical to accept help and support when it's offered. Not everyone wants to help or knows how to help. Take a step back to see who is in your life and is trying their best to support you to the best of their ability. Support is shown in many different ways. Appreciate these differences and accept help. Recognize that strong friendships last a lifetime and are hard to find. Embrace the people in your life that love you and are making an effort to reach out to you.

What is a friend?

"A friend is someone that you can be comfortable and uncomfortable with when you are confronted with the truth."
A friend will listen to you and support you, even when they don't want to hear what you have to say."

-Stephanie Rabi

"True friendship is about strength. It is someone you can safely tell all your secrets to without being judged, mocked or laughed at."

-Irina

"A definition of a friend to me is unconditional love. In other words sticking by them through the good and bad times and never judging them and always supporting them!"

-Cecila

"A friendship is the ability to put someone before you and to support, empower and encourage them to fulfill their unlimited possibilities."

-Amy

"A true friend will respect you when you want to be left alone, will sit with you in silence, will comfort you in need, will laugh with your not so funny jokes and will defend you in your absence."

-Janaki

Recap:

- Seek out the people in your life that have or can put a smile on your face and help you get off your emotional rollercoaster.
- Take time to interact with your family and friends. Go for walks, make dinner with your someone, or visit a place with them that triggers positive memories.
- Make a list of all the wonderful experiences that your family provided for you in your life and tell them how much it means to you.
- Call you friends and organize an "outing" to the mall, the movies, dinner, horseback riding, a concert or to meet and greet at Starbucks for lattes.

- Be open to meeting new people or rekindling a friendship that you have let lapse over the years. Creating change brings a feeling of shift and hope to your life, giving you something to build on.
- Rely less on online social networks to keep in touch with friends, as this isn't as powerful or healing as face-to-face contact. Make commitments to bond with friends through outings.

Chapter 3

Music

"I think music in itself is healing. It's an explosive expression of humanity. It's something we are all touched by. No matter what culture we're from, everyone loves music."

-Billy Joel

Ever since I can remember music has been an important part of my healing and happiness. Music is escapism. It is magical and celebrated on a universal level. A powerful form of communication that represents different parts of our lives. Everyone knows at least one song, band, style or beat of music that touches them deeply. Music has the power to inspire us and unconsciously lighten our moods. Studies show that it awakens the happy hormone dopamine and ignites our positive energy.

As a teacher I draw on music to teach my elementary students certain concepts, help them overcome shyness, build confidence, and express themselves.

As a little girl, I would lock myself in my room and dress up as divas Tina Turner, Madonna, or Cindy Lauper. I sang the lyrics out loud and felt alive, beautiful and creative. It was my escapism, yet it served a purpose for me later in life. Years later, I took my "show" on the road, lip syncing at grade seven and eight parties with friends. One time I rushed to Zellers for the latest tape cassette of Milli Vanilli so I could show it off and sing it with my friends at a party I would later attend. I was obsessed with watching the latest videos from Michael Jackson, Paula Abdul, Janet Jackson, and Madonna

In high school, my passion for music kept growing, and I participated in a school talent show with my friend Amy. We dressed up to perform a dance and then sang in front of the school. In grade nine, I began playing the drums. I am not sure how happy the boys in the high school band were about me being a drummer, but it made me feel alive. However, I did not continue with the drums simply because buying a drum set was too expensive and I doubt my parents would have appreciated me practicing at home. So, I ended up with a more sophisticated instrumented, the flute, which I played until I graduated.

My parents fueled my musical passion by bringing me to Broadway musicals such as Cats, Miss Saigon, Lion King, Phantom of the Opera, and The Sound of Music. This exposure gave me the confidence to try out for and obtain a small role in my high school production of West Side Story.

As I reached my twenties, I was going out every weekend to bars or local dances to sing, bond with girlfriends and dance until my feet hurt. University opened my eyes to the world of clubs, DJs, concerts, live music, and places to dance. My interests in different styles of music expanded and my lyric bank was growing and growing.

"Is there a song here you don't know?" I remember a friend once saying to me.

As I got older and was making more money, I attended concerts such as Madonna, Michael Buble, Blue Rodeo, Justin Timberlake, and Sarah McLaughlin. I visited local lounges and intimate venues to enjoy some of Toronto's local musicians and bands perform. Many of my favourite places for live music were—and still are—trendy jazz clubs and underground bars and cafes tucked away from Toronto's busy streets.

WHY Music?

Music is a natural healing medicine that alters emotions and moods. It is a form of escapism from our day-to-day reality. You can obtain music easily on the television, radio, computer, records, CDs, music stores, libraries, and from friends. You can make music from found objects, sticks, and make simple beats using your body, mouth, and vocal chords. Music is simple but affordable, attainable yet diverse. Within its beats, music contains healing powers. It is the music and the message that help us heal and lift our spirits.

Affirmations and Positive Messages

The month after my ex-husband left the house, I had found driving to work excruciating. Being alone with my negative thoughts haunted my mind. Each day I jumped into the car in agony, and noticed my anxiety was heightening. I dreaded driving to work and back again because I was totally alone, and could not call anyone to help me pass the time. At least at work, there were teachers and students around me to talk with and occupy my mind. It's not an exaggeration to say that music saved me from myself.

During this time I bought my first iPod and began downloading my favourite songs from iTunes and making my own playlists. I deliberately chose songs that gave me strength, hope, encouragement, joy and simply entertainment. Many songs spoke to me as though the singer or musician knew my exact situation. There were many songs at that time that I also just simply enjoyed listening to and that encouraged me to sing along.

Listening to my iPod everyday on the way to and from work, the music kept me company and kept my thoughts from straying into the darkness. Even though I was only distracted temporarily, those moments gave me hope. I sang as loud as I could, all the while tapping my hands on the steering wheel. Before I knew it I wasn't just listening to the music, but rather I was singing the lyrics and really absorbing the messages that gave me strength. My negatives were gradually transforming into positives. A big believer in positive affirmations—statements validating that something is true—I began believing in the power of affirmations after reading *You Can Heal Your Life* by Louise L. Hay. I took this book with me during my trip to Costa Rica and was able to find many affirmations to help me heal. It taught me the power that words have, and I am living proof that it works.

Friends, inspirational speakers, psychologists and counsellors often told me to look in the mirror and tell myself positive things. An example of this would be repeating to yourself "I love you," or "You are a kind person." I found this difficult to do on a daily basis considering how busy I am in the mornings and evenings; however, I was singing inspiring, life-affirming songs everyday and those songs contained messages and affirmations that I found easier to engage with. Singing these messages over and over was just another way of repeating daily affirmations.

Mood Boost

I like to think of music as my "mood booster injection." It was like being in therapy—only better! To go from feeling alone and unhappy, to lively and feeling content just by listening to music, is truly magical. Music was my companion through the most difficult times. Even if I only listened to it for a few minutes every day it transformed my spirits and allowed me to change the way I viewed my situation and my future.

I hated my long drives home because my negative and unhappy thoughts drove me crazy. My mind wandered, and I was continuously reminded that I was alone and dealing with the loss of my marriage. Even though I was able to focus my mind on the road, I still felt my mind wandering to hurtful memories that I was trying to forget. It was music that kept my mind concentrating on other things. I was able to focus on the lyrics and the messages of the music, so my mind did not have the time to remind me of the present pain. I was focused on singing the lyrics and predicting the beats, rhythms or lyrics.

I decided to take my music to another level to be more engaged in its power to transform. I asked my BFF to go out dancing as a means of "escape." This was my way of dealing with pain because being surrounded by funky lights, big crowds and upbeat music made me feel alive. I loved singing to the words and, similar to being in the car on my way to work, the music made me forget about my pain, and I was the only one who knew of my suffering. Surrounded by others I was forced to *hold it* together.

There were many Saturday nights with Stephanie dancing and singing until two in the morning, at which point we would then hobble home, our feet throbbing and our voices nearly gone. This feeling of liberation and positive expression soon became a part of our social routine. We would no sooner finish one weekend of dancing and singing when we would be planning the next. I remember that we even had our own songs that became tradition for us to listen to in the car before we arrived at our destinations. Stronger by Kelly Clarkson and Firework by Katie Perry were two of our favourites.

Katie Perry was my saviour through my difficult times because she had many songs that spoke to me. She was medicine for my pain and the anxiety. The songs *Firework* and *Part of Me* gave me strength and reassurance and it was as though she were speaking directly to me and my situation.

Firework

Do you ever feel like a plastic bag
drifting through the wind, wanting to start again?
Do you ever feel, feel so paper thin
Like a house of cards, one blow from caving in?

Do you ever feel already buried deep?
Six feet under screams, but no one seems to hear a
thing
Do you know that there's still a chance for you
'Cause there's a spark in you?

You just got to ignite the light and let it shine
Just own the night like the 4th of July

'Cause baby, you're a firework
Come on, show 'em what you're worth
Make 'em go, oh, oh, oh
As you shoot across the sky

Baby, you're a firework
Come on, let your collars burst
Make 'em go, oh, oh, oh
You're gonna leave 'em falling down

You don't have to feel like a waste of space
You're original, cannot be replaced
If you only knew what the future holds
After a hurricane comes a rainbow

Maybe you're reason why all the doors are closed
So you could open one that leads you to the perfect
road
Like a lightning bolt, your heart will blow
And when it's time, you'll know

The line, "You're original, cannot be replaced. If you only knew what the future hold, after a hurricane comes a rainbow" made me feel special. As I sang these simple lines to myself daily, I started to feel my confidence rising; the word "rainbow" in her song created a vision of light and new beginnings.

Part of Me

Days like this I want to drive away
Pack my bags and watch your shadow fade
You chewed me up and spit me out
Like I was poison in your mouth

You took my light
You drained me down
But that was then and this is now
Now look at me

This is the part of me
That you're never gonna ever take away from me, no
This is the part of me
That you're never gonna ever take away from me, no

Throw your sticks and your stones
Throw your bombs and your blows
But you're not gonna break my soul, this is the part of me
That you're never gonna ever take away from me, no

I just wanna throw my phone away
Find out who is really there for me
You ripped me off, your love was cheap
Was always tearing at the seams

I fell deep, you let me down
But that was then and this is now, now look at me

This is the part of me
That you're never gonna ever take away from me, no
This is the part of me
That you're never gonna ever take away from me, no

Throw your sticks and your stones
Throw your bombs and your blows

But you're not gonna break my soul, this is the part of
me
That you're never gonna ever take away from me, no

Now look at me I'm sparkling
A firework, a dancing flame
You won't ever put me out again
I'm glowin' oh whoa

So you can keep the diamond ring
It don't mean nothing anyway
In fact you can keep everything yeah, yeah
Except for me

This is the part of me
That you're never gonna ever take away from me, no
This is the part of me
That you're never gonna ever take away from me, no

Throw your sticks and your stones
Throw your bombs and your blows
But you're not gonna break my soul, this is the part of
me
That you're never gonna ever take away from me, no.

This was my "go to" song. Every morning without fail I
blared this song from my car speakers on my way to work. I
felt like my light had been taken, and I too had been chewed
up and spit out. She reminded me that no matter how bad it
gets or how bad the problem, I had to stay true to myself. My
spirit belonged to me. My spirit, and my soul would never be
taken. I realized I was special and that would never change.
This song also reminded me to be true to myself. Money,
personal belongings, revenge or resentment were things that
I slowly realized were not important to my happiness. I
began to focus more on who I was, and the type of person I
wanted to be and remain. Who is Sara Mody?

I did not want the emotional roller coaster I had been on for
several months to change me as a person. Sometimes, as I

was driving in the car, I would listen to the Katie Perry song and imagine that I was in my own music video singing directly to my ex and throwing my wedding ring in his face. This song overall, reminded me that no matter what had been taken from me and how much pain I was feeling, I was still myself and that being true to myself was MY CHOICE! It was the love that I had for myself to heal and move on with my life that became apparent through listening to this song. Thank you Katie Perry!

Recap:

- Write down the songs that make you sing, dance or simply put a smile of your face.
- Talk to friends or research bands that are making appearances in your city and check them out with a group of friends.
- Take some time to get out of the house and visit a local music store to enjoy the afternoon browsing through CD's, and checking out the New Release section for a popular band or singer.
- Treat yourself to a new iPod or music device that gives you endless access to music listening whenever you are feeling down and need a little lift.
- If you enjoy dancing but late night excursions are not your thing, perhaps registering for dance lessons such as ballet, ballroom, salsa or belly dancing will get you out of the house and enjoying different types of music.

Chapter 4

Health and Exercise

"To keep the body in good health is a duty... otherwise we shall not be able to keep our mind strong and clear."

-Buddha

I previously mentioned that during my marriage, I was diagnosed with breast cancer. After reflecting for days and researching alternative therapies to treat my illness, I decided to pursue natural treatments while undergoing a few medical recommendations from my oncologist. Looking back I'm convinced that fate brought me to Carol Morley, a naturopath working in my community.

After making the conscious decision to decline chemotherapy, I turned to her for support. She was my angel. Treating me with foods and supplements she not only helped me conquer my illness, but provided me with a safe haven to express my fears of dealing with cancer. Her office was decorated with inviting colours, and she had a positive personality that gave me confidence to try non-traditional methods. I was drawn to her warm smile and soothing eyes. What I remember most about my visit was leaving her office with a feeling of hope that I cannot explain. It can only be experienced. It is that powerful. Carol has a way with words. She makes you feel comfortable and powerful. On her recommendation I bought supplements, vitamins, fruits and nuts at my local health store. I owe much of my good health and love of food to Carol.

After months of following her diet and changing my lifestyle, I felt invincible and in control. When experiencing stresses in my life, I conjure up the "good feelings" I experienced when I met Carol, and how powerful I felt eating a balanced diet. She gave me hope, strength and supported my passion for food. Now five years in remission, I owe much of my strength and health to Carol. She not only had a hand in restoring my health during my battle with cancer, but she continued to influence me, and to help me heal.

The first three months of my separation had a huge impact on my health. It was apparent to my colleagues, friends, and family that my health was deteriorating, both emotionally and physically. The first few things that I experienced were lack of sleep and loss of appetite. Sleeping and eating are two of my favourite activities. I am a foodie. I love the taste, smell and experience of food. I get cravings for vegetarian pizzas, pastas, chocolate, warm buttered scones, salads, and soups. My social circle is usually surrounded by food in some form. I attend food festivals and farmers' markets, check out new and trendy restaurants, drive across town for a taste of gelato, buy cookbooks, grocery shop for healthy food, cook with friends, and enter food contests. Food surrounds me most of the time.

More importantly, everyone who knows me, is aware of how much I adore food and appreciate its health benefits. I owe my fight with cancer to food. It's the power of food that keeps me healthy and in remission. Yet, sometimes when tragedy strikes, you forget to take care of yourself and of what's most important. Consumed with pain and on the biggest emotional ride of my life I lost 15-20 pounds within four to six weeks and was popping sleeping pills nightly for months. I had lost zest and colour in my face. My eyes were tired and my skin was bleached with tears. For the first time in my life, I was finding clumps of my hair in the shower and in my hairbrush. At one point I stopped eating altogether.

Days turned into weeks and I was surviving on yogurt, bites of cheese and water. I did not crave my beloved chocolate, salads, pizzas or scones, which meant there had to be a problem. My friends were becoming concerned that I might actually fade away. Even my trip to Costa Rica was a partial waste since I wasn't eating the meals that were paid for in the all-inclusive package. As time went on, and I shed more weight, I was running out of clothes that fit properly. I stopped going to the gym because I was too weak and tired to do any of the classes. I was scared that I might actually faint or injure myself while working out.

The Power of Food

I remember coming home during the first few months of my separation and feeling alone as I entered the door and there was no one else there; no one to greet me with a hug and no smells of garlic or onion lingering in the air. I was alone and it felt strange. I had a life where I would come home to my husband and either he would have cooked a meal for us or we would cook together. Now, that was gone. I was on my own. Cooking intimidated me. I knew a few simple dishes but didn't push myself to learn more. Cooking for myself seemed lonely and tedious, and a chore. I was beginning to dread the idea of cooking for myself. I think deep down in my heart the thought of cooking by myself and eating reminded me just how lonely I was. I knew I had to find a way to change my thoughts about cooking and make it fun and make it mine. I had to own it.

One evening, hungry and not knowing what to eat, I stood at the entrance to my kitchen, staring at the stove and cookware I barely touched anymore, when the name Carol Morely came into my head. What would she think of me in this state? I was depriving my body of nutrition, which would eventually affect my ability to remain cancer-free. I needed to take charge.

"Sara, I know you are experiencing pain but you still have to fight to keep your cancer from coming back and you must stop doing this to yourself," I said to myself.

That evening I scoured my whole kitchen, rummaging through my cupboards and fridge to see what I had. I was disgusted to discover that I had no fruit or vegetables in the house. My bread was covered in mold and most of my dairy products had expired. Only a few boxes of grains and cans of soup in the cupboard remained. I began to pitch everything into a large garbage bag. I could not believe that someone who loved eating and took pride in her knowledge of health had such a pathetic pantry.

I grabbed my iPod and jumped in my car. I was on a mission.

At my favourite grocery store, I purchased nutritional food and food that was also delicious to me. Price was no concern. I filled my cart with organic vegetables and fruit, and decided to make healthy juices and smoothies with my juicer which I would have to dust off. I filled my cart with whole grain pastas, herbs, nuts, seeds, salmon, soups, lentils, almond milk, cereals, eggs, and of course, my dark chocolate. Just looking at the food excited me and made me feel better. As I started stocking my pantry with my new purchases, my full fridge began to inspire my soul.

I hear it time and time again, people making excuses for not cooking. I understand that everyone has his or her own reasons for not cooking. Many of my friends are married with children and time becomes their biggest challenge. It's difficult to carve time out for preparing meals and finding the energy to prepare and buy the ingredients. I am at an advantage because I do not have children. I only have two cats to feed and myself. I also heard the excuse that eating out at fast food places and restaurants is cheaper. I get that too.

I too have found that the prices in many grocery stores have increased and by the time you purchase all the ingredients and spices you need to make a meal you could have ordered it for half the cost. But cooking meals at home also creates leftover meals for other days. When it comes down to it, eating out will always be more expensive when you factor in that restaurants do charge more for a dish or appetizer, and then you add tax, tip, perhaps parking on top of that.

Take it from someone who loves eating out and trying different cuisines, cooking offers full control of what you are eating, and it saves money, builds confidence, and produces leftovers for other days. I think that there are different degrees of cooking but for the most part, if you can read, you can cook. Cooking does require a little bit of practice and a pinch of risk taking. On the whole, there is not much to reading a recipe, buying ingredients and following instructions. Finding healthy, delicious and fun meals to cook is part of the process and fun. There are so many resources available now to help you make meals that are nutritious and simple. Visit your local bookstore, or grocery store and you'll see all the resources that are out there to help you cook. The Internet is full of great cooking sides and links. The hardest part is selecting one to try.

Cooking was not only a positive distraction, but it also kept my emotions healthy and happy. I felt confident taking charge of the food that was going into my mouth and treating myself. As mentioned earlier, I lost about 15 pounds and then decided to take charge of my life and change the thoughts in my mind.

What kind of help would I be if I didn't share with you what I learned about food and its power, and the types of food that helped me through my emotional roller coaster? I am not a doctor, nutritionist or naturopathic practitioner. I am only sharing my knowledge about food and what I learned through reading in health magazines, websites, newspaper articles, and from other health literacy sources. Food and eating healthy are passions of mine and it is a lifestyle that I have chosen to live for me.

The following foods will not give you instant gratification or cure your depression but they are a step in the right direction. Everyone is different and will experience different results of pleasure and happiness. I do believe that a "healthy person is a happy person." So let's get you started!

Yo! Yo! – Greek Yogurt

When I was going through my depression I was literally living off of yogurt and Greek yogurt. Yogurt has many benefits. It's high in calcium and protein, and is easy to store, eat, and mix with other foods to create amazing dishes. Yogurt is a super on-the-go snack when you feel down and need a lift. Greek yogurt can be used in shakes, baking, cooking and dips. My favourite way of eating Greek yogurt is to add it to a smoothie. It's easy to make and easy to take on the go. If you've been depressed and aren't eating much, it's also a super way to slowly introduce your stomach to digesting food again while also putting nutrition back into your body.

Recipe with Greek Yogurt: Banana and Strawberry Smoothie

- 6 ounces Greek yogurt or flavoured (i.e., blueberry, strawberry)
- 1 banana
- 4 frozen strawberries
- 1/4 cup cold water
- 4 ice cubes
- walnuts
- 1 tablespoon peanut butter or 2 tablespoons hemp seeds

Blend all ingredients together.

Chocolate

Ever since I was a little girl, I have loved chocolate. My mother not only always had it around the house, but she exposed me to foreign chocolates. Being Scottish, my mother opened my world to loving the extensive selections of UK chocolate. I grew up loving chocolate digestive and orange Club biscuits, Lion and Penguin bars, Jafa cakes that were delicious if you dunked them in hot tea, British Smarties, and my personal favourite, Cadburys.

I remember eyeballing the chocolates that were so generously dumped into my pillowcase every Halloween. Believe it not, I kept a running inventory of the flavours and number of chocolate bars in my candy stash. I knew how many Kit Kats or Oh Henry! were in my sack as I went door to door in the night. When I got home, I was never surprised to see my mother rooting through my stash for safe candy and to get a sneak peak at my chocolate. I never minded sharing it with her because I knew she loved chocolate as much as I did. We have always bonded over chocolate at birthdays, dinners, holiday celebrations, difficult times, or just sharing a bar while we waited in line at the grocery store.

However, the type of chocolate to help you with your health and your depression is not milk chocolate, but rather dark chocolate. This type of chocolate raises the chemicals in your brain, such as endorphins, which lead to a state of euphoria. Now, I am not saying to go out and eat a few large dark chocolate bars and all your problems will melt away. What I am saying is that a few pieces of this magical dark treat will put a smile on your face and help you to think positively.

Recipe with Dark Chocolate: Poached Ginger Pear with Chocolate Drizzle

Ingredients

- 4 to 6 fresh pears
- chopped fresh ginger
- 2 tablespoons honey
- handful of Hershey's Dark Chocolate or Purdy's Dark Chocolate bars

Directions

1. Slice piece off bottom of pears to make a flat base. Peel pears and core from bottom but leave stems intact.

2. Combine ginger and honey in a saucepan of boiling water; add pears, base side down after the water as boiled. Boil pears in saucepan for about 10 minutes; reduce heat. Cover; simmer, spooning juice over pears occasionally, 10 minutes or until pears are tender.

3. Remove wrappers from chocolates; break into smaller pieces. Place chocolate pieces in small microwave-safe bowl. Microwave at medium for 30 seconds and stir. If necessary, microwave an additional 10 seconds at a time, stirring after each heating, until chocolate is melted when stirred. Or melt chocolate in a different dry pan until melted.

4. Place pears on individual serving plates; drizzle with melted chocolate. Serve immediately. Makes 4 to 6 servings.

Go Fish and other Omega Nuts

Foods like salmon, tuna, mackerel, flaxseeds, walnuts, and pecans are rich in omega-3s, and as such have incredible anti-inflammatory benefits. But, that's not all. These powerful nutrients can actually change your brain chemistry and help to alter your thoughts. Practising good nutrition by taking omega-3s naturally via your food is just one more way for you to produce positive thoughts and prevent depression from taking hold.

I have been exposed to fish all my life as my father loved seafood. Family trips to Florida were my personal time to enjoy fresh seafood and connect with my father. Through him I came to appreciate oysters, mussels, escargot, lobster, crab, salmon, and shrimp. We would stop at restaurants along the way to stuff our faces full of some sort of wonderful ocean food. Even now, when I visit my parents, I know my father will probably serve garlic escargot before dinner, shrimp in a pasta dish, or salmon with a Dijon mustard glaze.

During days when I felt really sad and could not pull myself out of my negative thinking, I made sure to eat something that contained omega-3s. Even grabbing a handful of nuts in the morning on my way out the door contributed to keeping my dark thoughts at bay.

If you really do not like the taste, smell or texture of fish or have a nut allergy, there is the option of taking omega oil.

Greek Salmon Salad Penne

- 12 ounces whole wheat penne pasta
- 3 tablespoons extra virgin olive oil
- 1 yellow bell pepper, cut into ½ inch strips
- 1 15-ounce can of chick peas
- ½ cup pitted kalamata olives
- 4 garlic cloves
- ¼ teaspoon red pepper flakes
- 5 cups baby arugula
- ground pepper and salt to taste
- 1 to 2 salmon filets
- ¾ cup feta cheese

Prepare the pasta according to package directions, omitting any salt or fat. In a large bowl and reserve ½ cup cooking water to drain. Bake the salmon and add to pasta. Heat oil in large pot over medium heat, add bell peppers and cook for 3 minutes. Add the chickpeas, garlic, red pepper flakes. Combine the remaining ingredients, except for the feta. Refrigerate for at least an hour, up to overnight. Add feta.

Kale—My Green of Choice

For an instant pick-me-up when you're feeling low, try eating leafy greens, cheese, eggs, meat, seafood, beets, beans or lentils. Loaded with beneficial B vitamins, they fight stress and can help with anxiety. Spinach, kale, Swiss chard and broccoli, are all green veggies that protect the delicate membranes around brain cells, and prevent negative thoughts from appearing.

Think of these healthy foods as a fortress around your brain cells that protects against depression, anxiety and negative thoughts. When battling my cancer, kale was my knight in shining armour. I believed that it helped me fight my illness and grow stronger.

In Carol Morley's book, *Delicious Detox*, her recipe for kale chips became my go-to snack to make during my separation. I munched on them on my long drives home from work, and, unlike potato chips, the nutrients in this super food helped me focus on happy thoughts. As I mentioned previously, driving home was one of the most difficult things about my day. Every time I jumped in the car my heart would sink knowing that I would be alone. The kale chips were one of the healing medicines that got me through my illness, also through my depression.

Kale Chips*

- 1 bunch of kale
- 1 tablespoon extra- virgin olive oil
- 1 teaspoon sea salt (a pinch of red chili flakes is an option too)

1. Preheat the oven to 375 F

2. Remove the stems from the kale.

3. Wash and dry the leaves and tear into bite-sized pieces.

4. Drizzle the leaves with the olive oil but remember to use little oil because kale chips will shrink.

5. Line a baking sheet with parchment paper and place the kale leaves on top.

6. Bake in the oven for 10-15 minutes until the edges are brown, but not burnt.

*From Carol Morley's cookbook, *Delicious Detox*

My Kale Salad Recipe

To a large bowl of ripped kale add:

- ¼ cup olive oil and massage oil into the kale for 3 to 5 minutes or until it softens
- ½ squeezed lemon and 1 tablespoon lemon zest
- handful of sunflower seeds, walnuts or pecans
- parmesan or blue cheese
- diced apple (bite-sized pieces)
- drizzle of balsamic vinegar
- pinch of salt
- 2 cloves of chopped garlic

Green Tea

I am in LOVE with green tea! During my fight with breast cancer and during my depression, this tiny leaf was my health buddy. In fact green tea from my local Starbucks was my drink of choice while writing this book. Green tea contains thiamine, a substance which is said to help you relax and focus. That must be why I drank endless cups while working on this book. Green tea kept me focused enough to get my thoughts and ideas down on paper, while at the same time keeping me in a positive mood. When I wasn't in Starbuck's writing and drinking tea, I would often take a trip to David's Tea to load up on my favourite green teas. A Canadian company, David's Tea has many stores across Canada and the United States, and serves about 150 different flavours of tea that will satisfy anyone's taste.

If you don't like drinking green tea yet wish to experience its healing properties, just make a pot of green tea and pour into ice cube trays to freeze for cold drinks.

No matter what, I always have colourful fruits in my fridge such as blueberries, strawberries, raspberries, oranges, grapefruit, pomegranates, and pears for recharging my body systems and altering a bad mood. We've all heard that an apple a day keeps the doctor away. Fruit contains fibre, vitamin C, folate or folic acid, and potassium. It lowers cholesterol, is relatively low in calories and helps prevent health complications such as high blood pressure. Fruit is also the food I reach for when I need a boost. Trust me, when I say that eating a handful of raspberries or blueberries will alter your energy and put a smile on your face. Fruit is colourful, has citrusy scents, and is bursting with sweetness.

Exercise

Any form of exercise can help with depression and help build confidence. You may choose to exercise at a nearby gym, your local community centre, at home, or with a friend. Regardless of what activity suits you the best, the important thing is to find something you like and to commit to it. The key is to stay active! Don't worry if you don't have something in mind right away as finding something you enjoy takes time. Keep in mind that exercising with a friend will keep you continuously active because it creates accountability and motivation. A workout buddy will keep you focused and ultimately make it fun and enjoyable.

Here are a few types of exercise that you can do alone or with a buddy.

- running
- yoga
- golfing
- dancing (i.e., "Just Dance" videos on YouTube).
- gardening
- housework, especially sweeping, mopping, or vacuuming
- jogging at a moderate pace
- skipping
- joining a sports team (i.e., volleyball, soccer, baseball, basketball)
- walking

Because strong social support is important for those who experience depression or big life changes, joining a group exercise class may be beneficial. Exercising with a friend will help you benefit from the physical activity and also the emotional comfort, knowing that you're being supported.

Once I felt determined to take control of my health, everything fell into place. I religiously went to the gym four to five times a week, and began running on community trails four times a week after work. I replaced coming home from work and taking sleeping pills to changing into my running gear and grabbing my tunes. I started enjoying smoothies and protein shakes and eating healthy dinners again. I dined out a few times a week to experience different ethnic foods and eat at trendy restaurants that I had always wanted to experience. I felt alive and rejuvenated. I was enjoying eating again and during my slow process of introducing food back into my life, I had not noticed that I was sleeping without tears or taking sleeping pills. Colour returned to my cheeks and my energy was coming back. People frequently told me I was glowing. These positive comments made me smile and kept me going because I felt that if others were noticing, and taking to time to share their thoughts with me, that I must be doing something right. My experiences are described below. You don't have to copy them but instead use them as examples of how you can create your own experiences.

Yoga

Yoga is a form of disciplined exercise that originated in India. It offers benefits to the body both physically and mentally, and spiritually. Yoga's goal is to attain a state of permanent peace. While running and dancing boosted my energy level and gave me a feeling of accomplishment, yoga helped me reduce stress and tension in my body. Through breathing exercises and mediation, it allowed me to release negative thoughts and feelings. I found it difficult at the end of the yoga class to sit quietly with my thoughts and meditate for ten minutes. Yet, in time I was able to do it.

Mediation to me simply means a state of peace and clearing the mind of all conscious thoughts. It is a process where you de-clutter the mind of stresses and worries and allow it to become empty and at peace. Studies show that meditation can lower blood pressure, depression, anxiety and other healthy issues whether mentally, physically or emotionally. I encourage those I know to try meditating for three to five minutes every day. Allowing some time everyday to clear the mind of stresses is beneficial to overall health no matter how it is accomplished.

Previously I spent countless hours trying to distract my thoughts of hurt and wasn't allowing my mind to deal with reality. The distractions were only temporary and my pain wasn't going away. I went to my yoga class for the first time in months after my ex-husband left. As I struggled through planks, sit-ups, bends and warrior poses, I began to feel strong and in control of my thoughts. Though my thoughts didn't run away from me during the class, the meditation at the end scared me. I was afraid my thoughts would wander and my emotions would conjure up something unpleasant. I knew I would not be able to focus on my breathing and concentrate on relaxing.

As I lay on my mat in the dark, in a peaceful yoga studio, I listened to my instructor's words about relaxation and escapism. My mind couldn't focus properly on her voice for more than a few moments without being pulled to think of my situation and my fears. Tears welled in my eyes and down my cheeks. I didn't feel embarrassed or intimated to allow tears to fall since it was dark and everyone around me had their eyes closed. Mine were open and staring at the ceiling. Like a dog pulling a leash, my mind kept pulling me deeper and deeper into my trauma and loneliness. I finally surrendered, allowing my mind to take its course. It needed and wanted to get these memories out, and so it was my mind using meditation as its outlet, its way to escape. It took about two months of daily meditation before I was able to meditate again without crying and feeling sad. Having gone through every memory stored in the brain, the mind had released each one into the universe for me to never dwell upon again.

Running

When I was younger I used to run sporadically and never really stuck with it. Instead of sitting in my empty house, I decided to get outdoors and enjoy nature. There is a gorgeous trail that runs from my place, through the woods, along streams and flourishing nature. Many walkers and bikers used this trail all year round so I knew it was safe. Every day, I found the energy and determination to put on my running clothes and grab my trusty iPod. The first few weeks were extra-difficult as I was constantly gasping for breath and having to stop along the way. At the beginning I felt that maybe running wasn't for me when I started realizing that something else was actually happening.

It became another chunk in my day when I wasn't thinking about my pain or about my failed marriage and broken heart. It was another period in time when I wasn't crying and feeling down about myself. I loved being close to nature. I was breathing in the fresh air, listening to my upbeat tunes, feeling the sun on my face (of course while wearing my sun block!) and smiling at passersby. I decided that I had to stick with it. The overall health benefits like toning and building my endurance and the simple enjoyment of getting out of the house and being one with nature were enough to encourage me to continue. I was becoming addicted to feeling free again and running was making me feel good about myself. I would sing along to the songs that empowered me and could feel my body becoming stronger and stronger.

It's a proven fact that exercise improves moods and decreases side effects in conditions such as menopause. As an example, my oncologist recommended I participate in physical activity everyday to diminish menopausal symptoms I was experiencing while on my medications for cancer. Regular exercise was increasing my energy level while allowing me to benefit from the feeling of being tired after an invigorating workout. As a result I was sleeping deeper and longer, and waking up feeling refreshed.

Of course part of feeling good after exercising was due to the increase in endorphins, which decrease the intensity of pain in individuals. Not only do endorphins act as a pain regulator but they are said to be connected to physiological processes including euphoric feelings, appetite modulation, and the release of sex hormones. What I found interesting while researching endorphins is that there's a term "runners high" that captures this feeling of euphoria and of what happens when endorphins are produced and released due to exercise.

Another thing that I'm certain produced euphoria in me was being in nature while running. There, I was able to connect with trees and see their beauty. Also, at the end of my run, I would hug this large tree and remind myself that I made it through another day. While focusing on myself and loving me, it was during one of these moments immersed in nature when I decided to get a tree tattoo. A tattoo of a tree would represent my *new* beginning, and the branches would represent possibilities that my life was experiencing. Trees are very important to me, and the symbol of a tree reminds me of my magical journey, and the beauty of nature.

Golfing was another activity that I decided to explore. It's funny that I chose this particular sport because golf has always been my father's favourite sport to play. He lives, eats and breaths, golf. I think growing up I hated golf simply because I felt that I was constantly competing for my father's attention when it came to golf. If he was not playing golf every weekend, then he was barging into the family room, grabbing the television controller and changing the channel, from whatever I was watching, to GOLF.

As a little girl, I knew that if I couldn't think of what to buy him for Christmas, his birthday or for Father's Day, I could always buy him either golf balls or golf shirts. When I was growing up, he often wanted me to golf with him, or take lessons. Yet, it never really interested me. That is until recently. Strange how major changes in life can alter one's perception. I inherited a set of golf clubs from my sister and purchased some golfing outfits during one of my visits to Arizona. One day the cold weather and my dark depression forced me to throw my clubs in my car and head to an indoor driving range near my home. I found a spot where there was no one else around, and after hitting a few balls I felt liberated yet also scared. My father had given me a few introductory lessons on *driving* the ball, but mostly I had no idea what I was doing. What I did know was how to keep my eye on the ball at all times and how to swing.

I spent an hour-and-a-half shooting balls into the distance, and, for a few moments my mind was free from the hurt. I was out in public, golfing in the middle of February, and releasing my tension and aggression into a tiny ball and knocking it away with gusto. Golfing became my visual symbol. I visualized my anger, my ex's face, my resentment and my pain, sitting on that tee. Hitting that ball with all of my strength and all my might, and watching it fly through the air, gave me satisfaction I cannot explain. I felt free. Golf gave me an outlet for my frustrations and another opportunity to build my confidence while keeping my mind off my sorrows.

Golfing also gave me the opportunity to spend quality time with my father during that difficult summer after my separation. I enjoyed loading the car with our clubs and golfing shoes. Even though I was a beginner, I felt like a pro in my matching pink shorts and golfing shirt. I listened to my father with pride and love while he coached me on posture, stroke and techniques that he had learned over the years. He made me smile inside. Once again, I felt a tranquil state wash over me as I basked in the sun and walked the course with my father. I began to build confidence in myself as a golfer when my father would praise me for shots that were successful. At the same time, I was patting my own back for finding a hobby that was fun and relaxing, even, or especially one that I had despised most of my life. Golfing gave me an outlet, an escape, and a chance to connect with my father, and to learn a challenging recreational activity.

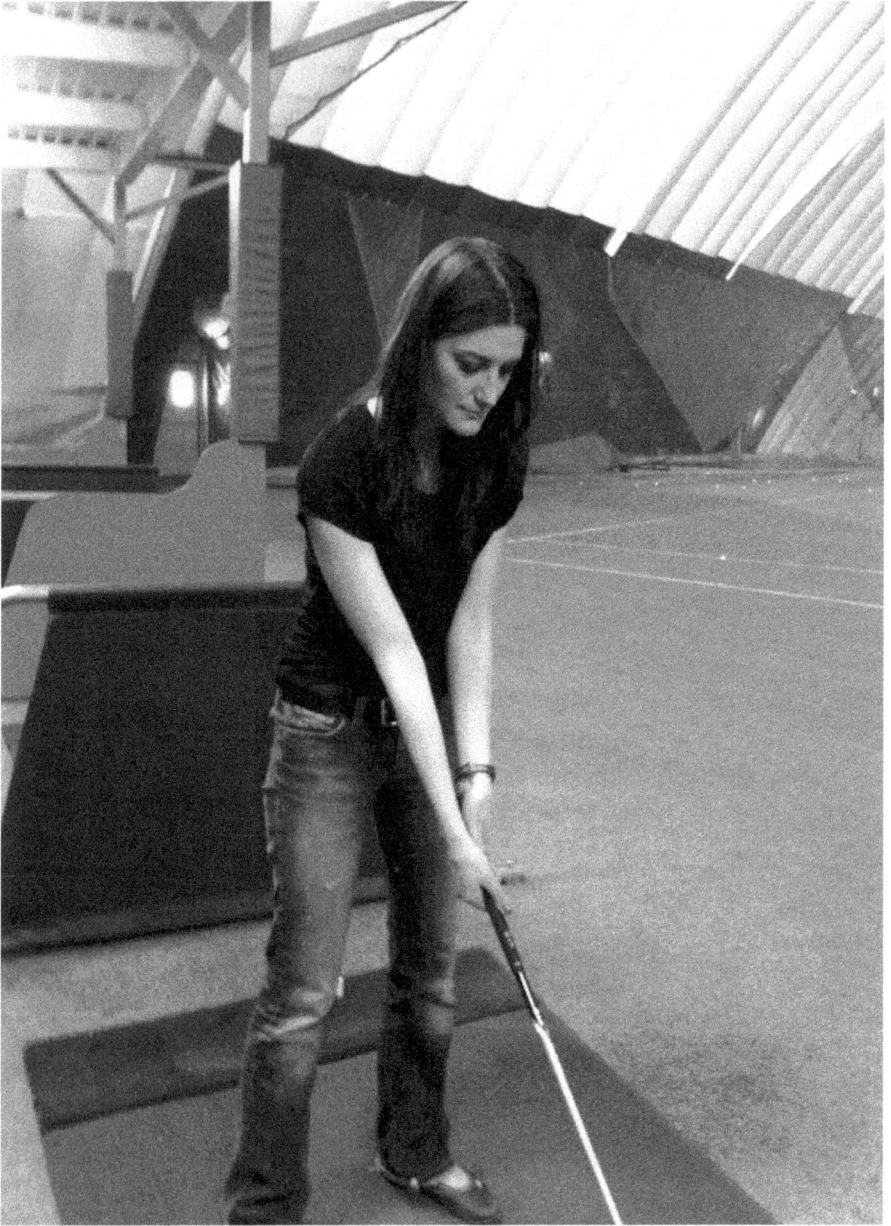

Rediscovering a Hobby

Recap: It's up to you!

Diet

- Take a moment to reflect on the foods you eat.
- Keep a food journal of what you eat each day and make space to write down areas where you can make changes to incorporate better eating habits.
- Plan a day in your week to spend some quality time at a favourite grocery store. Invest in healthy foods to stock in your kitchen.
- De-clutter your kitchen of junk food, pop and sugary treats and organize it in a way that inspires you to spend time there cooking and eating healthy.
- Find ONE recipe that you would love to try and spend a night cooking, while sipping wine and listening to music. Better yet, invite a friend over to help you and then you can both enjoy the meal and each other's company.

Exercise

- Go for a walk, run, or bike ride.
- Do yoga in the park.
- Take up a new activity to try out with a friend or family member such as golf, kayaking, tennis, or join a soccer recreational league.
- Run a marathon for charity.
- Join a local gym. Gyms are a great way to meet people, promote health and fitness, and keep yourself busy.

Chapter 5

Passions and Hobbies

"Hobbies are like flowers on a plant. They make the plant look beautiful and feel proud."

-Sukant Ratnakar

Passions and hobbies are the pots of gold at the end of the rainbow. They help us better ourselves, meet people, expand our experiences, open doors, build our confidence, and add value to our lives. Everyone should have some hobbies. You might think a few are too many, but I think that having more than one is healthy. Your hobbies tell a story about the type of person you are and who you wish to become.

When going on dates or meeting new people, you often hear, "What sort of things do you like to do?" or "Tell me something about yourself?" Hobbies help us discover who we are and guide us to find out more about ourselves. Meeting someone who has many hobbies tells me that this person is open, experimental, has goals, and enjoys challenges. In some ways, a hobby defines who you are as a person. For example, while going through the following list of my hobbies, see if you can paint a picture of the type of person I am. I love painting, yoga, cooking, reading, shopping, dancing, golfing, listening to music, gardening, writing, art museums, travelling, and watching old movies. Any guesses?

There is a difference between hobbies and passions. One can have many different hobbies for enjoyment, or experimental and learning purposes. Hobbies can change, yet a passion is more constant and can motivate success, action, and accomplishment. Passion is powerful and takes precedence over everything else because you feel and think about it constantly. A hobby can lead you on a journey to success. A passion typically starts out as a hobby. I believe that everyone has a deep, inner passion they want to explore. A passion lingers in the back of the mind waiting to be discovered. It will exist and grow stronger until it is acknowledged, embraced, and explored.

Whatever dreams you want to turn into reality are your PASSIONS. The old saying, "You can do anything if you put your mind to it," is a simple but true statement. Believe in your passions. Ask yourself what you dream about doing with your life? What makes you happy, and what do you find yourself talking about with the people who are close to you? If you had a free day to spend doing something and money wasn't an issue, what would you do with it? Pay attention to your responses and you might find your inner passion. Both hobbies and passions are gateways to self-discovery. Hobbies begin the journey of discovering activities that you may or may not be interested in, and eventually one or more can become passions and lead to self-discovery.

Hobbies not only expand our experiences but also allow us to meet new people. If you don't engage in any activities or have any interests, it makes it difficult when contributing to conversations with other people. As an example, when I talk with someone new, I can tell that person about my travelling adventures and places I have visited. That leads to other topics about things I have seen or enjoyed. From there, the conversation can take off in unexpected and interesting directions.

Hobbies are investments in your being. They offer opportunities for you to learn about yourself and discover hidden talents. As mentioned before, my parents are my role models and they have exposed me to the joys of life. Growing up I was given the recreational activities. My father and mother both supported and believed in extra-curricular experiences. As a small child, I remember going to camps, and being involved in swimming, cooking, drumming lessons, modelling, ballet, tennis and many others that interested me. I never felt like my parents were trying to keep me out of trouble as a teen. It was more that they wanted me to try new things and broaden my interests. Even today, I had a conversation on the phone with my mother about being busy with my writing, my painting, my yoga, and taking a makeup course. As usual, my mother supported me and listened to me with an attentive ear as I spoke about my hobbies.

During my separation, painting became a new hobby for me. I'm not sure exactly where my interested came from because I had never painted in the past. Before investing in supplies, I decided to take a few painting courses to make sure that I enjoyed painting. After completing an introductory painting course and completing my first piece, I fell in love with how painting made me feel. It was tranquil, artistic, and therapeutic and allowed me to not only escape from my sadness but also left me with a finished product that made me feel proud.

Painting in the park became my summer outlet with my friend Amy. My favourite day was visiting a park near her home and setting up near a stream. We had packed our painting kits and a picnic. I remember feeling the sun on my face and the fresh air fill my lungs like a helium balloon. She and I spent almost four hours that day conversing, laughing, snacking and covering each other with splashes of acrylic paint. Many bystanders or observers stopped to watch us and engage as we continued to apply paint to our canvases. Similar to exercising and listening to music, painting became an escape from my pain and negative thoughts. It was a bonus to share this hobby with my friend and enjoy spending time with her.

Another activity that became a passion after my marriage fell apart was writing. Ever since I can remember I have loved the world of literacy. How could I have avoided it? My mother was a teacher and a public school librarian. Books surrounded me most of my life, and growing up I participated in writing contests. I recall one of my high school teachers giving me a disappointing mark in my last year of high school, and I had to repeat the course. I was mortified to show my mother this mark and felt like a failure. I did not understand how I could love reading and writing so much and barely pass. I repeated the course with another teacher, William Bell, a renowned author of young adults novels. Now, the pressure was on.

I admired this teacher's dedication, knowledge and openness to teaching literacy. He inspired me to work hard and to love writing even more. He is one of the role models in my life that planted the seed in my head as a teenager, that I wanted to one day publish a book. He gave me hope that I could do anything if I wanted it badly enough. Mr. Bell, if you ever read this book, thank-you for believing in me.

As the years went by, I knew I wanted to publish a book, but I never knew exactly what I wanted to write about. I took a poetry course in university and thought that maybe I could publish a book including all my poems. That lasted about a year and I scrapped that idea. Next, I took a course on how to write and publish a children's book. I dreamt and plotted about this for two years before my chicken scratches of ideas found their way to the garbage. Even though I had fallen in love with children's stories and storybooks, writing one was not my calling. The curiosity was there but not the drive. Next, I took a seminar on writing cookbooks. This project still lingers in mind every day. When I was diagnosed with cancer, I finally thought I had found my idea for the book that I was meant to write and share with the world. I could write about my journey battling cancer. I attempted many times to sit down and record my experiences, but it never really captured my heart. There were so many books and resources available that I never had the confidence that my story was worth telling. I wanted a book idea that was different, positive and unique.

Writing about separation became my calling. This journey was the story that I felt I needed to tell and share. It was my personal story. The doors of writing opened up to me as I began journaling and sharing my stories with others. It became very clear to me like the sun shining through the mist that I had a book to write that would help others and give them hope. My separation was not an easy one or an amicable one. Quite the opposite. Yet I survived and my life flourished in so many ways.

Spending Sundays in Starbucks on my laptop, I was inspired and dedicated to complete my book and have it published. It was my passion. My calling is now to share my story with women and give them support, inspiration and hope that they could make a difference in their own lives. Not only that, but that they could also survive a separation or another heart-wrenching hurdle that might come their way.

We all have stories to tell and experiences to share. Writing is now not only my passion but also my destiny. Every time I felt sad, lonely, or had lost hope to deal with my situation, I would jump in my car and head to Starbucks to surround myself with people and bask in my love of writing and love of words. I love to spend my time relaxing with my journals and pen and watching my thoughts and emotions come to life. Publishing a book has always been a dream of mine. Keeping busy with this project has given me focus, built my confidence, and helped me to deal with my pain.

One afternoon, while sitting in Starbucks on a rainy Saturday, sipping a delicious latte and nibbling on soft banana bread, a thought crossed my mind. What if I never publish my book? What if no one ever reads my book and I cannot help someone heal? That made me think that maybe I was wasting my time. Obviously my end goal was to publish this book and put all my long hard hours and money spent on lattes to good use. Then I smiled. I remembered that this book was created out of the simple concept that journaling was therapeutic and helped me a great deal to heal during my depression. The writing was put to good use and was crucial in my healing process. My end goal was to engage in activities that brought me peace and confidence. That made me happy and helped me to grow as an individual. Writing this book has taught me so much about myself, my friends, talents, interests, and strengths. More importantly it has shown me that I can do anything I want to do if I put my mind to it. I can achieve my goals.

Writing this book has forced me to reflect on all of the positive things that I have done for myself to help me heal and become a stronger person. I am strong. I am talented. I am important. I have a voice and wonderful stories to share with the world. So do you!

Hobbies show us who we are and who we want to become, whether we become published, noticed, or a professional guitarist, dancer, singer or cook; it is remembering a simple philosophy. I use this same rule when I am teaching children art in my classroom I am not concerned with the end product. What is important to me is their process. What did they learn and how did the activity stir their emotions along the way? So my advice is to find a passion that makes you happy and brings you peace. You can do it!

Hobbies open doors for us to meet and spend time with others. Hobbies facilitate interaction with other people who share common interests and allow for fun or educational conversations. I constantly find myself using the expression to myself and to others, "You won't experience life sitting on your couch." This statement holds so much truth for me. When I think of this statement, it inspires and challenges me to find out who I am and to enjoy all that the world has to offer "by doing." Getting out into the world and embracing it, experiencing it, and opening myself up to it is the only way to feel truly alive. Simply put, hobbies allow growth and learning and will enable you to flourish.

I have met some of my closest friends in places such as the gym, a course, a workshop or a festival. You are meeting people that you share common interests with and you begin to bond with people as you interact. It's easy to connect with people who share similar opinions and interests. By involving yourself in recreational activities, you open doors to the possibilities of meeting new people and to becoming engaged in new experiences. Opportunities do not come knocking on your door. They are created and explored. They are out there waiting for you to discover them.

Most memorable events in my life started off with a simple hobby that opened doors for me and led to amazing things. My most favourite memory started as a hobby and led to memorable experiences.

There is an event in Stratford, Ontario called the Savoury Culinary Festival. It happens every year and I had always meant to attend. Amy and I shared a passion for food and for cooking, and I knew I wanted to experience this event with her. I knew Amy and I would enjoy eating food and bonding, and that I could meet Canadian Chef Vikram Vij, one of my favourite Canadian chefs. He owns two world-renowned restaurants in Vancouver—Vij's and Rangoli and was going to be at the Stratford Festival doing cooking demonstrations. Amy and I drove through a torrential downpour all the way, which didn't stop the two of us laughing and making the most of a messy situation. When we arrived in Stratford, we were too late and had missed Vikram's presentation. I was extremely disappointed but decided to forget about it and enjoy our time together. Amy promised to make it up to me.

Two days later, she called me on a Monday and told me that she had two tickets to a breast cancer event called Cook for the Cure, where five Canadian Chefs would be present, including Vikram Vij. She assured me that tonight I would meet him. Overwhelmed with excitement I rushed home to take a shower and then headed back downtown. I was not going to meet Vikram sitting on my couch.

When I arrived, I saw him chatting away with people, and I began building my courage to walk towards him and introduce myself. Finally after two glasses of wine, I knew it was now or never. It was my reason for being there that evening, and I had to just go for it. I walked up to him, stuck out my hand and told him of my disappointment not seeing him in Stratford, my background, my love for food, my story of breast cancer and before I knew it, he had invited Amy and me out for a drink after the fundraiser event. The events that followed, as miraculous as they seemed to me, simply unfolded in a natural and beautiful manner.

One evening I met him for dinner to discuss my goals, my book, and ways I could raise money to attend the Cook for the Cure event. He was inspired by my story battling breast cancer and wanted me to cook on his team. It was a cooking showdown event to raise money for breast cancer. Definitely my type of fundraiser. Participants got to cook with a Canadian chef and build points to create the best menu with some predetermined ingredients. At the same time, the event raised money for breast cancer research. I felt overwhelming gratitude as I reflected on what was happening to me. Here I was, meeting, conversing, sharing and learning from a

Canadian culinary idol of mine and having the good fortune to cook alongside him. Thinking back I knew that if I hadn't pushed myself to walk up to him and share my story, I wouldn't be living my dream and discovering who I was—and am. My hobby and passion had led me to my dream of cooking and learning alongside a master.

Months later, Vikram Vij came to my school and helped me to fundraise the money I needed to cook alongside of him. Parents, students, friends, and family all generously donated money to my cause, and before long I had raised the money. One month later, I was at the Fairmount Royal Hotel with sheer gratitude in my heart and anticipation running through my body. With the help of students, friends, family and coworkers, I had reached my goal of $2,500. I was fulfilling my dream of cooking alongside Vikram and having the chance to learn from other Canadian chefs such as Mark McEwen, Chuck Hughes, and Corbin Tomaszeski. I was meeting all kinds of amazing people, getting my picture taken, supporting research for breast cancer, eating delicious food and having the opportunity to be interviewed by Global and City TV. I walked away that night a changed woman with the smells, flavours, discussions, human warmth and laughter firmly planted in my memory. Not to mention, Vikram and I are friends, and I cherish that very much, and admire his humble attitude and warm heart.

Having cooking as a hobby and finding pleasure in food brought me to become a participant in the Cook for the Cure, making it to the top 50 fundraisers in the event. I took a chance to raise the money because I had a passion for cooking, for the world of food, and an interest in getting to know local chefs. The activities that led up to that night at the Fairmont Royal York Hotel were possible because I took my hobby a little further.

But that's not all.

A year later, at one of the launch parties for the Cook for the Cure 2014, I approached a Canadian Breast Cancer Foundation (CBCF) employee. It was similar to the event I had attended where I had met Vikram. I told her I was interested in helping the CBCF by sharing my story with breast cancer at any upcoming events that she might have in the future. I told her that I was interested in building my public speaking experience and I wanted to give back. I was surprised when she told me that she would keep my name on file and let me know if anything came up. A few months later, once again I was totally surprised when she contacted me to see if I would be a guest speaker for the CBCF at an upcoming Cook for the Cure launch party, featuring Vikram Vij.

I felt so honoured that she trusted me to speak in front of an audience and genuinely happy that I could share my story. There is nothing more I enjoy in this world than sharing stories with others. I have never been afraid of public speaking or reading stories to others. After all, I am a teacher. My every day is reading stories and listening to stories from children and other educators. This event was an exciting experience and opportunity for me. I never imagined being a part of this experience and sharing my struggles with fighting cancer and sharing it in a positive way. Once again, something new and unique was happening to me. I was constantly seizing the moments and challenging myself to become a part of events all around me. It was a world I would not have imagined for myself two years ago when I was undergoing pain and feelings of hopelessness.

"I am participating in the Cook for Cure Culinary Showdown because I recently met a young lady, named Sara Mody, who was diagnosed with breast cancer at a young age. What is interesting about her story is that she turned down chemotherapy treatment and made the decision to fight her cancer with the healing powers of food. She has used the art of "Auyurveda", which is eating healthy and using spices like turmeric, ginger, garlic, cumin, and cloves. These amazing spices are a huge part of my style of cooking and my heritage. Sara has been fighting her cancer with food, meditation, yoga, laughter and positive thinking. She will be reaching her five-year cancer-free mark in February 2014. At present, she is feeling alive, strong, proud and grateful. Cancer has become a positive part of her life, because it has taught her about herself and how to live; the attributes that are necessary in life to keep strong and remain focused. The experience has become a vital part of what makes Sara, SARA!"

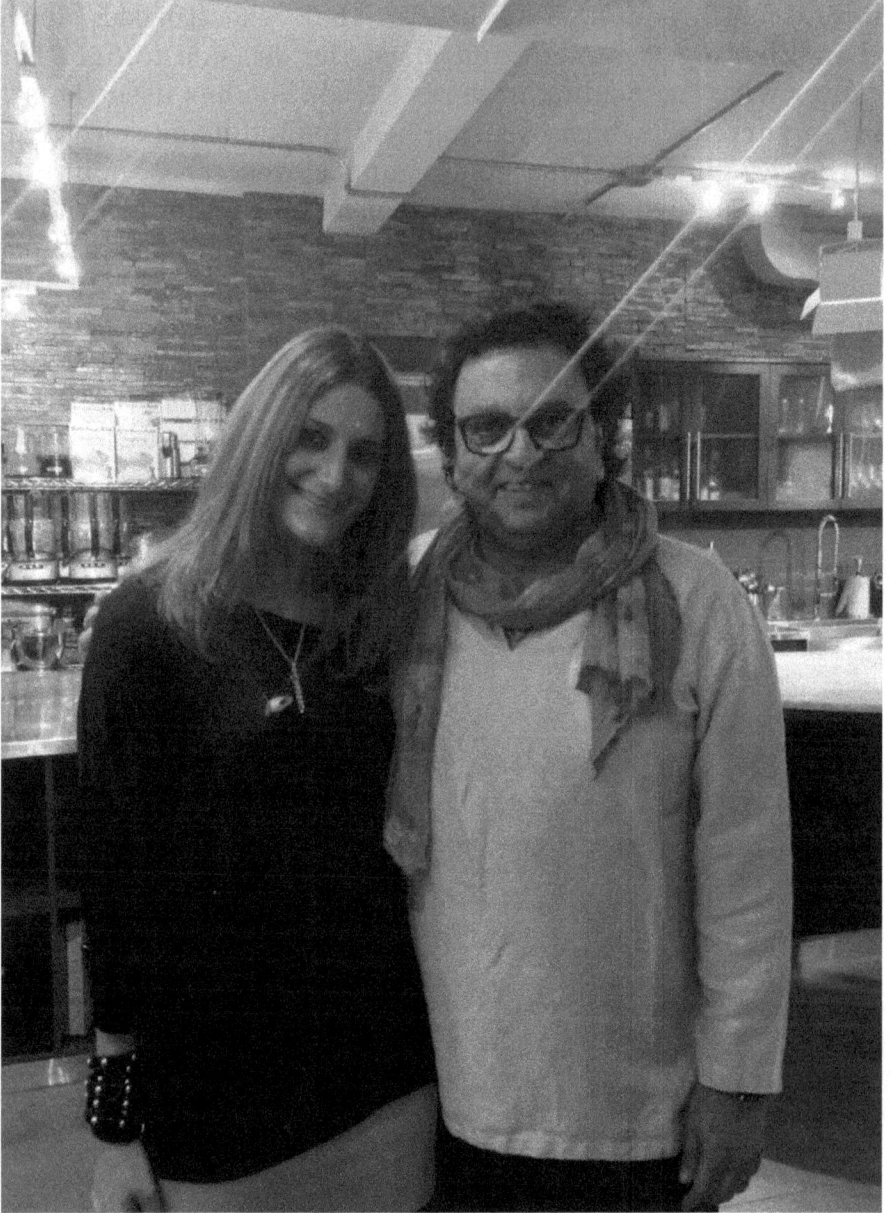

Vikram Vij and I

Sara is a huge fan of Indian cooking, being half Indian herself. It will be a dream come true for us to cook together and showcase our cuisine and culture on December 7th in

Toronto for the Cook for the Cure event. It will be especially meaningful for Sara to be a part of this event as a survivor who has used food as her medicine and has joie de vivre attitude in life.

http://www.foodnetwork.ca/blogs/HostsandInterviews/2013/1 1/14/Why-Vikram-Vij-is-Cooking-for-the-Cure/?id=69529

Meeting Alex at Cook for the Cure

At the same event, I also had the privilege of meeting a young man named Alex. I was wearing a chef's jacket that was given to participants to wear during the cooking portion of the event. Turns out the jackets were donated by his company, Chef Works, in Canada. After hearing my story and learning how I managed to raise the money for breast cancer, he offered to make me my very own pink personalized chef's jacket. The jacket has the breast cancer ribbon on the left hand side and the words Canadian Breast Cancer Foundation underneath. After receiving my jacket from Alex, a friendship evolved, and together we came up with a concept of using my pink chef's jacket to visit restaurants together. I wore the "Travelling Jacket" to restaurants that we wanted to eat at and I got my picture taken with the jacket, in the chef's kitchen. Every time I wear the jacket I am spreading awareness for the cause and sharing my story. Then I write about the restaurant on my blog. Together, Alex and I enjoy tasting and talking about food. I am grateful for meeting him and for having the opportunity to share our mutual passion for food.

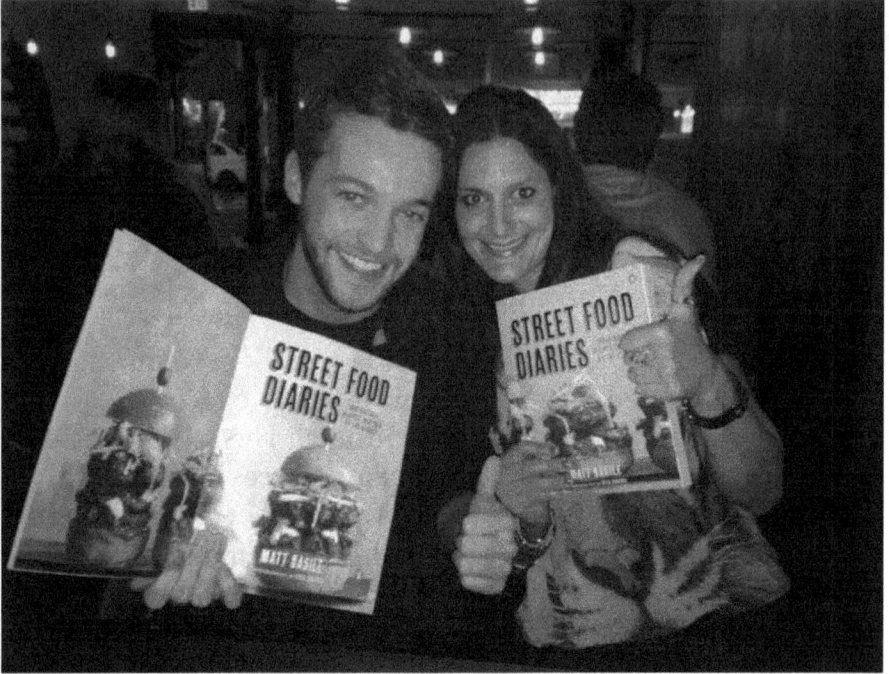

Alex and I at Lisa Maria

He is a kind, fun and loving friend.

Being a part of Cook for the Cure was a wonderful experience that I will never forget. The food, excitement, celebrity chefs are all elements of the night that make it memorable; however, the friends that I made that night are the most meaningful to me, and I can continue to build new experiences with them.

"Attended the Canadian Breast Cancer Foundation KitchenAid Canada Cook for the Cure fundraiser and met this inspirational lady cooking on Vikram Vij's team. She was the happiest I saw there all night and she had a great story to tell as she had suffered with breast cancer and chose to take the route of eating her way through it making good choices and refused any chemo to treat it. When she met her idol Vikram who inspired her to eat well and when he heard her story he told her she must attend! This event takes a lot of fundraising to even participate however and she did not think she could. Vikram came to her school where she teaches grade one students and held an entire assembly there! He spoke of many things and asked for everyone to donate what they could. After many days of students grateful enough to contribute even loonies and toonies she eventually had enough and was able to join his team and cook for us that evening! She was beautiful on the inside and out and takes joys in the little things in life. You can learn a lot from talking with a person."

-Alex Argiropoulos

A year later, I was asked to share my inspirational story of Cook for the Cure and my battles with breast cancer at another launch event. I was to speak in front of possible fundraisers for their chance to support the cause, raise money and participate in the culinary cook-off of the year. Vikram would be there too, sharing his story, and my friend Alex would be there supporting me. It was a wonderful honour and I felt I had purpose to help and inspire others while sharing my story. At this event, I had the wonderful pleasure of meeting Brooke Feldman, a recent participant in the 2013 Master Chef Canada series. I instantly clicked with her and we exchanged numbers. Brooke is an inspiring, open and courageous young woman. She has a culinary talent and a dream to take her cooking passions to another level. Since then I have had the honour of attending restaurants, spiritual conferences and meditation classes with her. She has taught me many things and inspires me to do better every day and reach for the stars.

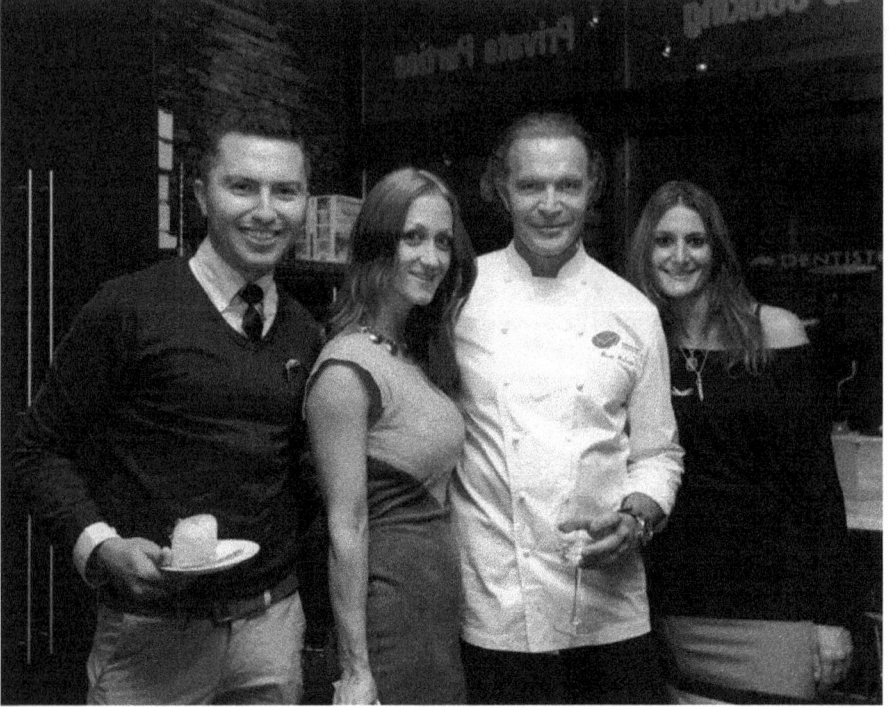

Fouad, Amy, Mark McEwan, and I at Cook for the Cure

Recap:

- Make a list of all the things that you like, even if it is sounds silly or irrelevant. Finding links between the activities you like might lead you to the right one.
- If you already have a hobby, then set aside time in your busy week to explore it.
- Write your hobby down on a calendar or post-it note so that you allocate time to it.
- Research programs or events at local community centres, libraries, city recreational programs, or online sites such as Meetup, Facebook or Twitter for ideas and events to become involved in or to give you ideas for what to pursue.

- Ask your friends what sorts of activities they are presently involved with or would like to try out with you.
- Organize your own club around a hobby such as food, film or books where you watch films with others, check out a new restaurant, or meet to discuss novels you've read.

Chapter 6

Cry

"Crying represents the best and worst of what it means to be truly alive."

-Jeffery A Kottler

I would be lying if I said I didn't cry. In fact, after the breakup with my ex husband, I cried often. Often is an understatement for the crying that actually occurred. During the first few months, I think crying was all I did. It felt like a disease taking over my body. I had a hard time sleeping, talking, thinking, driving, and simply existing without shedding buckets of tears. Sometimes, I cried because I was crying too much. I cried in the morning, at work, after work, in the car, in the shower, to any song I heard that reminded me of my failed marriage, or anytime I was alone with my thoughts.

Crying became a part of my daily routine. I quickly learned to anticipate and accept it. One night as I lay in bed I remember wondering when the crying would end and if I would ever go a day without blowing my nose? I wanted the ability to move on. My outbursts were taking over, and I felt wretched and out of control every time tears began to form.

I noticed patterns to my crying. Driving, mornings, waking up and lying down to sleep were the worst. These were the moments where "crying" became a natural form of expression for me. It reminded me that I was not moving on with my life.

One Saturday night I was coming home late from Amy's house. I remember leaving her home and challenging myself to make it home without shedding a tear. I turned up the music, focusing on the fun I had that night and how grateful I was for having supportive friends. About half way home, my heart once again broke, my concentration wandered and tears began to roll down my cheeks. My eyesight blurred and I tried to compose myself as it was late at night, and I didn't want to cause an accident. Then without realizing it, I sped through an intersection making a left hand turn. Immediately following, flashing lights appeared behind me. I tried to compose myself and took many deep breaths, hoping the officer wouldn't notice my wet rat look. When he approached my window, he asked me why I was speeding. I apologized explaining I was upset because my husband was not coming home and I was thinking he was having an affair.

The cop smiled at me and said, "Things will start looking up." Then he told me to, drive safely and have a good night. I thanked him, took a deep breath and went on my way. I later told Stephanie about the incident and she and I laughed when she shared a similar story with me.

Getting stopped by the policeman reminded me once again that I was not moving on. I wondered if I would ever heal and move forward.

Sleep was my other problem. I had trouble settling in bed because of uncontrollable outbursts that interrupted my sleeping. It was hard for me to relax and drift into sleep. Instead, I would lay in bed, pondering my life, and my depressing situation over and over again. I even tried crying myself to sleep but that never seemed to work. It was my mother's suggestion that perhaps I should consider sleeping pills temporarily, so I could function during the day. I took her advice and was finally able to rest.

My mother and father could not bear to listen to their daughter's sobbing from their spare room every weekend when I visited. The sounds of my crying chipped away at my father's heart and he would beg me to stop. He felt helpless in the face of my pain, and it really weighed down on him. I felt comfortable crying in my parents' home. I felt loved, supported and at peace crying alone in the spare room. The girl they had raised to be confident, happy and successful was like a shipwrecked soul. I was taking them with me on an emotional roller coaster. They wanted desperately to help me heal, yet they also wanted to get off.

Throughout this book I have encouraged you to try new things and to push yourself because I also want you to heal and know that eventually you will move on to a brighter and more beautiful future. I am not advocating that every day you plaster a smile on your face, cook an exotic dish, run a marathon and mingle with strangers while ignoring your true basic instinct, which may be to cry and release. On the contrary, I am encouraging you to release your pain by crying as much and as often as you need to. Crying is a natural part of healing. Accepting your pain and "owning it" will help you move on and heal. Only when you accept your pain can accept yourself. Self-acceptance helps you to avoid putting yourself down and moves you in the direction of building your confidence. It prevents you from feelings that are NOT moving on. Many people I have spoken to expressed to me that crying means a person is weak and is not moving on. Yet quite the opposite is true.

Crying is a critical part of your healing, and so you must remember to embrace every moment and allow yourself to cry. I created the following statement to remind me it was good to cry:

"The more you cry, the less you will." I strongly believe that crying represents strength and bravery. By allowing yourself to cry, you are accepting that you are vulnerable and are not in control. You are strong enough to accept the most raw part of yourself and possibly share that vulnerability with someone else. If you prevent yourself from crying, then you neglect what your body naturally wants to express, which are emotions that will eventually explode into your life at another time.

Crying helps you bond with those near to you. It allows you to open yourself up and become vulnerable with friends and family that love you. Your true friends, as mentioned earlier, will love and support you and allow you to express yourself. It is your friends and family that will attempt to find solutions to make you smile and laugh. Your friends and family will be there to help you pick up the pieces. They are the ones you can count on to come over with buckets of ice cream, chocolate, wine, and movies to watch with you and keep you company. These little acts of kindness are creating beautiful bonds with your friends. There is something amazing occurring when you open up to your friends with pain and sorrow, and they understand and support your hurt. They pass you the tissue boxes and listen attentively. They hug you and constantly give you words of encouragement and hope that you want so desperately to hear. They sometimes even take on your pain for you; however, while they do accept that you are sad, they also don't want to see you continue to cry because they hate seeing you suffer.

And so they find ways to help you smile. Work on trying to keep your mind and heart distracted. I know that distractions are my best weapon for fighting my pain, anger, or depression. When I am around my friends and family doing exciting or new things, I temporarily forget my current situation. My waterworks dry up and joy and laughter fill my soul. It is a wonderful feeling to experience true acts of kindness demonstrated by friends and family going out of their way to bring joy into your life.

Many of my friends would take me out for a night on the town, buying me a full-bodied glass of red. Or they would take me shopping Saturday afternoons and then to the movies for a comedy and to pig out on popcorn. Because my parents remember me as an infant, a toddler, a young adult and a teenager, they try to help by saying things that are familiar to them or that have worked in the past. Regardless of what they suggest, it is their effort that makes it meaningful.

What are tears? To me, tears are a visual representation of your most organic feeling. Jeffery A. Kottler describes tears as a metaphor for human feeling. He believes that tears tell the world about us on a personal level. In his book, "No More Tears", he explains that tears have different purposes. They are a form of communication and are occurring for a purpose. Kottler contends that it's important to reflect on our tears and question what they are saying? According to him it is critical to trust yourself and your emotions as you surrender to letting go.

One of his theories that resonated with me is when he refers to holding back on crying as "emotional constipation." I loved this analogy. We do not want to suppress our emotions because emotions are naturally designed to be expressed. He comments on how suppressing crying can lead to health issues such as insomnia, digestive problems, and stress on the body. Crying is the body's way of releasing stress.

"Crying is an experience that comes upon us," writes Kottler, "rather than something we just do." We don't usually make the decision to be out with our friends and plan a moment in the evening when we are going to cry. In fact, for the most part, we try avoiding situations or conflicts that might lead us to crying. Yet in spite of this, crying often picks the most inconvenient times in our lives to surface. It creeps upon us without us having the strength to hold back. Kottler believes that tears are a powerful force. There are no rules or reasons to why we cry and how often it occurs. Crying is its own entity. All you can do is accept it and allow it to take its course.

Eventually, my crying did slowly come to a halt. It took time, but one day it just vanished without me realizing. I chose to work every day during my separation even though many suggested I should take time off. I am not the sort of person that works well with little or no distraction. Distractions give me strength, and being around children, curious and full of energy, all day long gave my mind something else to focus on. Oh, I did cry daily at work for several weeks but composed myself during teaching. I am a professional and even though there was sadness in my eyes, I did not cry around my students. I had the support of colleagues who would bend over backwards to support me and give me breaks during the day to help me cope. I had administrative duties, parents, photocopying, lessons, twenty grade ones, report cards, and so on, to keep me busy all day. Yet, at the back of my mind was the dreaded thought of not wanting the bell to ring, as that would mean my busy day was over, and I would have to dismiss my students and walk back to my empty classroom without their little voices asking me for help or their laughter filling my ears.

Children's laughter is one of the most beautiful and pure sounds and I needed to hear it more than ever before. The sound of silence in my classroom told me that I was alone and had to go home to an empty house. During those first months I would routinely sit behind my desk and cry my eyes out. Teachers walking by could not see my weakness as I was hidden in the privacy of my classroom. This behaviour repeated itself for months until, one day, it just stopped. Little by little, I was healing and moving on.

My well of tears was diminishing as was my pain, and I was getting my life back again.

It's funny how during this time of transition, specific days and the feelings I had on those days seem so clear to me. For instance, there was my birthday weekend when I got gussied up in a knock 'em dead sequined dress to go out with my best girlfriends. Dancing through the night, I had a perpetual grin on my face and sincere laughter—not tears—emanating from my heart. I previously mentioned how much I loved dancing. When I dance I am transported to another place. My laughter that night was organic and real.

That doesn't mean that I did not sometimes have moments when I reminisced about my broken marriage, and felt loss and sadness, I did. I still called Stephanie or my mother to vent or cry and hear their reassurances; however, I have learned to accept these moments. Each time, I have a tiny breakdown, I tell myself that my tears are a reminder that I am a human with a heart and soul. I accept myself for who I am: A woman with a large heart who gives herself completely to everything she does and to everyone she knows. What can I say...I love to love.

Crying has taught me so many things about myself and about the power of self-acceptance. The old Sara would have believed crying was negative and a sign of weakness, that crying represented pain. I had never reflected on crying until I was on the emotional roller coaster of my marriage that ended and had begun my journey of reflection and healing. I now know that crying is a gateway to emotional resolve and the body's way of dealing with emotion, whether happy or sad.

Think of it this way: We cry when we laugh too hard and we cry when a friend gives us a sincere compliment that we find overwhelming. We cry when we are having a bad day and we become frustrated. We cry when a song or a smell reminds us of a memory that we had forgotten from our past. Crying is a part of who we are and we learned to do it A LOT from when we were infants.

As children, we bawled our eyes out when we didn't get our way with our parents, or when we were teenagers dealing with the raging hormones from puberty, dating and not making it on the cheerleading or baseball team. Crying is an act of expression we would share with our best friend under blankets and clutching buckets of rocky road ice cream and soggy tissues. Somewhere along the way, we have forgotten to embrace crying and look at it as something positive.

So please allow yourself to cry. Trust me if you don't cry now, it will show up later!

"I think crying is important. Crying is a way to express your feelings just like yelling or laughing. It's important to express your feelings and not keep them bottled up. Crying is not a sign of weakness. Showing emotions makes you stronger because you are actually feeling."

-Natalie Knezevic

Recap:

- Accept your crying. Listen to your body and don't allow anyone to tell you to STOP! Remember crying means you are moving on! The more you cry, the less you will.
- Release one night to your friends and family and be open to any suggestions that your friends might have

to help you smile. Remember your friends want to see you smile and it would make them feel good to know that you appreciate their efforts.

- Find a moment in the day or the week when you can sit alone with your thoughts and allow the tears to come out. Remember the more you cry, the less you will need to eventually.
- When you begin to notice that your crying occurs less often, make sure you praise yourself.
- Write down a list of things that make you happy and bring you pleasure. My list consisted of chocolate, Yuk Yuk's Comedy Club, shopping, yoga, painting, dancing, and spending time with my friends. These were my "laughter distractions" that I resorted to when I felt like I was crying too much and needed a helping hand to get me out of the rut.

Chapter 7

Travel

"Travel is more than the seeing of sights; it is a change that goes on, deep and permanent in the ideas of living."

-Mary Ritter Beard

There is no price on the experience gained from venturing outside your familiar environment. Travelling is extremely powerful. When you travel, you gain gifts that enhance your life. There is not one single person in the world that does not have somewhere in their mind they would like to see or experience. Most have a natural curiosity for something different, exotic, mysterious or peaceful.

Travel represents release, escapism, romance, beauty, and knowledge. I feel it's important for everyone at some point, if possible, to plan a trip somewhere in the world to experience the unknown. Why do I feel so strongly about this? Well, because travelling forces us to open our minds, change our perspectives, gain knowledge, and it allows us to experience life outside of our own comfort zone. You do not need to travel far, just somewhere you have not been before no matter how close by.

I am fortunate to have been able to travel. My father's job involved travelling and he was constantly collecting travelling points. My mother was a school teacher and always had holidays and summers off for trips. Most of my memories and experiences are related to travel. I have been fortunate enough to experience India, Scotland, Ireland,

Spain, Italy, Holland, Belgium, Portugal, St. Lucia, Costa Rica, Bahamas, Bermuda, Newfoundland, Boston, Arizona, Serbia, Bosnia, Croatia, Montenegro, Paris, Turkey, Germany, and the Czech Republic. Even so, I still have many more places on my bucket list. There were two places in particular that I was blessed to visit and that helped me heal. One is Costa Rica and the other, Spain.

It was a cold, grey December and my marriage was quickly disintegrating. I had so many questions, yet no answers were forthcoming. At that point, I still had a husband, yet he wasn't communicating with me. I now know that he was actually in the process of leaving me without telling me that another women had replaced me. I spent endless nights alone in my house with emotions of anxiety and uncertainty welling up as I began to expect the worse. I came to a point where I knew there was no hope of making my marriage work. The absolute worst part was not hearing honest answers from him. Alone in my uncertainty, I started to accept the words separation and divorce, even though, he was not telling me what had changed and why. I felt lost, confused, sick, and completely depressed.

At the same time, I was still visiting Sunnybrook hospital for my cancer check-ups, tests and blood work. Alone. To top it off, it was Christmas, my favourite holiday of the year, and I was spending it without my husband. A home filled with memories of Christmas music, decorations, presents for each other under the illuminated tree, mugs of hot chocolate at our sides, and laughter wafting through the air. Yet that Christmas there was none of that. The home felt gloomy, empty and uninviting. The only thing I could stomach assembling was a small optical fibre Christmas tree. Over the holidays I would curl up on the couch and stare at it for hours as I tried to make sense of what had happened and come to terms with the fact that my marriage was ending. I hated Christmas that year. I purposely avoided watching my favourite Christmas movies. Even the commercials made me cry. My favourite part of Christmas had been shopping for gifts for my husband's stocking. Now I wasn't even sure if I should buy him something and the thought of giving him something knowing that he was leaving made me angry beyond description. As the fateful day drew nearer, my anxiety to get out of that house and see my parents began to grow. I just wanted Christmas to arrive so that it could be over. I wanted my holidays to begin so I could rush home and spend time with my family and have them support me like I knew I desperately needed.

Costa Rica

One evening my sister called to say that she thought I needed a trip. She recommended that we go to Costa Rica together for the holidays. I had never travelled with her before and the thought instantly eased the anxiety that had been building up since my breakup. An exotic trip with my sister gave me a positive distraction from my chaotic inner world and also gave me something to look forward to. I have always admired my sister's strength and patience and was really looking forward to spending quality time with her. As soon as she said I needed to go away with her, I knew instantly that she was right. I would stop thinking about how lonely I was feeling, and instead make new memories with those I loved and who loved me back.

I don't remember the journey to Tambor, but I recall waking up the next morning in the hotel and feeling different. Costa Rica is a place of organic beauty. The people were so warm, and the lush forests, exotic wildlife and beautiful beaches instantly lifted my spirits. My sister and I went zip lining in the tropical rainforest canopy, and, ATVing past pristine beaches and amongst the tallest trees I'd ever set eyes on. We relaxed in natural hot springs, drinking wine and listening to wild monkeys in the distance. Costa Rica is where I met JC, the wonderful tour guide who not only showed my sister and me around the countryside, but also took the time to talk to me about my situation and give me advice. To this day we still keep in touch through Facebook, and I will always remember how he made my sister and I laugh.

Costa Rica is the place where I meditated on the beach to clear my mind of negative thoughts. Every day I would sit on the beach and stare at the ocean for answers. It only took a few moments before tears rolled down my cheeks, and my thoughts got the better of me. Reality and acceptance kept creeping into my thoughts. I knew that when I left Costa Rica, my life was going to change for good. I was certain that I would return strong and willing to make the necessary changes in order to continue accepting my separation and healing. Being alone with my pain forced me to face my dark thoughts, accept them, and move forward.

Memories can be very interesting and powerful. I remember the very moment I felt alive, free, and at peace while in Costa Rica. I have a distinct memory of crying all morning and feeling self pity. My sister treated me to an ATVing adventure for the afternoon because she believed that was what I needed. I recall straddling the huge vehicle and stepping on the gas. I felt intimidated by the large machine but excited.

My sister was right behind me as we sped through bushes, beach sand, thick forests and dusty roads. I decided screaming with laughter was better than admitting just how scared I was driving the massive machine. I was terrified of falling and injuring myself; however, I felt more free than I'd felt for a long time as dirt splattered across my face and wind ripped through my hair. This was not the moment to feel sad or to ponder my failed marriage. I had so much adrenaline boiling in my blood that I was on a high. In that moment it was hard to feel unhappy. I felt grateful and proud for picking myself up and trying something different. I knew at that moment, this trip was only going to get better. I had hope in myself that I was going to heal and be happy.

My sister and I spent New Year's Eve in Costa Rica laughing in the hotel room as we listened to Rihanna songs. The next day we went zip lining in Monteverde and witnessed the finest cloud forest canopies in the country suspended about 100 feet up in the air. Costa Rica is where I sat in natural hot springs, saw exotic wildlife, and tasted the finest coffee. When I left Costa Rica after one week, I felt as though I had left my emotional baggage there and was filling my life with new memories. You can do the same anywhere that suits you. The action, activity, and emotion is more important than the location.

Before going away to Costa Rica, I began reading "How to Heal Yourself," by Louise Hay. I decided to take the book with me along with my journal. My first goal for the trip was to find peace and end my crying. My second goal was to bond with my sister, and my last goal was to finish this book and find something within its pages to help me heal!

On January 9th, shortly after getting back from Costa Rica, I wrote in my journal,

"Well I didn't cry when I got up this morning. I am proud of myself. I can do it. I am strong and deserve to be loved. I am grateful for my family, health, friends, and my job."

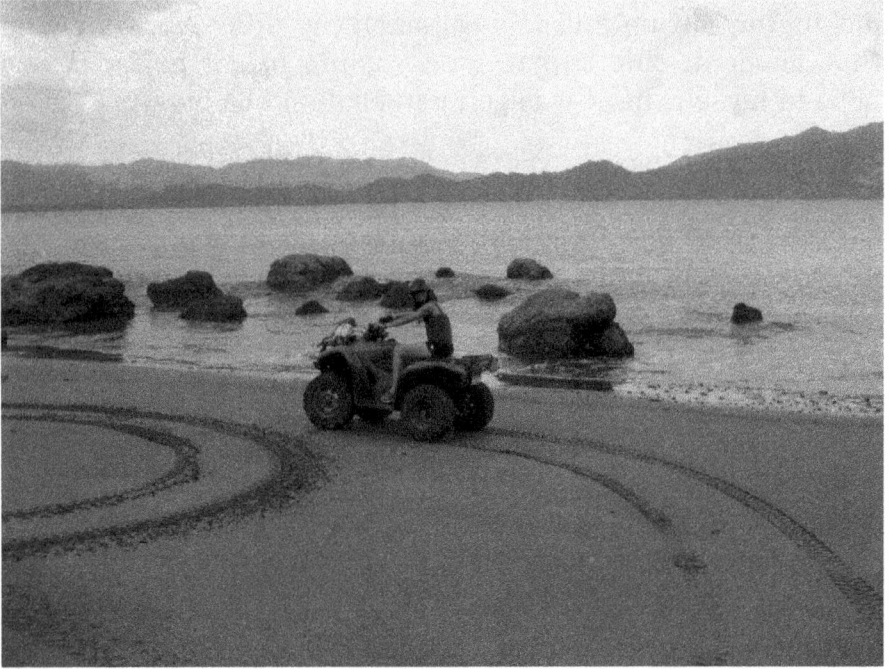

Me in Costa Rica

Spain

Several months after my mind-blowing trip to Costa Rica, I was already planning my next trip this time with my friend, Irina. She had suggested that we take off to SPAIN! Since I had such an amazing time in Costa Rica, I knew another trip with another willing participant would bring me even further along on my healing journey.

I visited Spain a little over seven months into my separation. My legal papers, including possession of the house, were not yet finalized, but I was in a happier, healthier phase in my life. I was finally living again! Spain was the trip that taught me about MYSELF. It was the country where I found myself and reflected on the riches of my life. And I don't mean financially. When I speak of riches, I am referring to my experiences, my job, my health, my family, and my friends. It is the country where I recognized how grateful I was for all the "positives" in my life. I brought my journal to Spain and recorded the experiences that I learned, saw, and felt. You can do the same.

On July 13th, I soared over the ocean to an exotic land. Being an avid writer, my journal and passport were the two items I needed to pack in my carry on. Hours after we departed Pearson International Airport, I was sitting on the plane with my pen and journal in hand. This is what I wrote:

"Well, I am on a plane on my way to Spain. I am so excited to see what adventures lay ahead. Irina sleeps beside me. I am so lucky to have her in my life. I never imagined when I met her that I would be on a plane with her to Europe. Sitting here, I realize how important strong, loving, supportive friends are. Life is a big adventure and I am blessed to have such amazing friends to walk with me on this journey."

Once we landed our adventures started immediately. We got lost finding our accommodations, we drank too much Sangria on a patio and ended up in a tapas bar eating olives and sardines. We spent the next morning sightseeing the streets of Madrid. We ventured on trains, subways, and taxis experiencing the sights and sounds of Barcelona.

One day, I spent a few hours alone in a café on La Rambla sipping cappuccino and snacking on soft chocolate croissants. I became preoccupied with people watching as hundreds of tourists passed in front of my table. I zoned out for a few moments soaking up the sounds of Spanish music, the smells of baked goods, and the sights of people going about their daily lives. At that moment all I could think about was, "I am in Spain. I am in Spain. This is amazing. I cannot believe I am actually here." After everything I'd been through, it felt surreal. I pulled out my journal and began recording the thoughts going through my mind at that moment. I wanted to preserve the memory to revisit it later. This is the spot and the moment where I decided that I should fulfill my dream and write a book. I wanted to share this moment with the world. I wished I could bottle up all the positive energy I had experienced and hand it out to anyone that felt that there was no hope of repairing their broken heart. Laughter snuck up on me and I quietly giggled to myself. I was feeling an overwhelming aura of gratitude.

July 18, 2012

"I am sitting at a cappuccino bar in Barcelona. I am writing in my journal while drinking espresso and reflecting on how lucky I am. I am so grateful for life, for my friends who love me, and my family who supported me. Sara, look at how far you have come in your separation journey. You have waited eight months for this journey to end. Eight months of tears, stress, pain, anxiety, uncertainty, confusion, betrayal, sadness, and struggle to have this moment of laughter. To be happy. To be free. Be grateful. Be yourself. Live again! Live again! Live again!"

It was also on this day that I decided to call my book Wide Awake because I felt that I was finally seeing clearly the type of marriage I had, and the type of relationship I truly desired and deserved. Not to mention, I listened to Katie Perry's song Wide Awake every day. One of my all-time dreams was to meet her and thank her personally for writing inspiring, strong, and empowering music.

Spain elicited an independent and adventurous woman inside of me. I needed a place to release and overcome my weaknesses and insecurities. It was the place where I discovered the meaning of true friendship. Spain is the journey where I began my new life and became a new person. The memories that surround this trip will remain with me forever. I will never forget the joy of snacking on warm pastries and cups of rich coffee every morning. Irina and I ate at cozy tapas bars drinking Sangria in restaurants that claimed to have the "best Sangria." My memories of dancing until six in the morning and meeting Spanish men on the cobblestone streets made us feel like we were supermodels. Irina and I ate the best gelato, listened to Spanish guitarists, and experienced buskers at every turn. I saw gorgeous historical landmarks such as Gaudi's, Sagrada Familia and walked the streets of La Ramblas. I cruised inviting boutiques, ate delicious churros, and tasted my very first authentic paella.

On top of all the wonderful memories I have from Spain to me the most critical was finding myself while challenging myself; I learned that I am a strong, open-minded, and positive person. I felt alive and began to believe in myself once more. Having restored faith in myself showed me that I was moving down a path of self-discovery and new beginnings.

This trip made me realize that I wanted to travel more. This trip allowed me to realize that if I had not gone through the heartache of a separation and was not on my own, I would have not travelled to Spain. Even if I had gone to Spain with my ex-husband, then the trip itself would have been a totally different experience and I would have not learned the art of being grateful. I wanted to make gratitude a part of my every day routine. I understood that being on my own was an opportunity for me to travel, experience and grow. I have always travelled and loved travelling; however, now I was travelling for myself. I was not with my parents or my ex-husband. I was travelling where I wanted to go and feeling free to truly embrace every moment.

There is not one thing that I did not fall in love with while visiting stunning Spain. I was able to see Madrid and Barcelona, and I think I left my heart in that country. I adored the food, the music, the people, the weather, the culture, the architecture, the history, the tapas bars, the festivals, the clothing, the wine, and the overall energy and aura of the country. Barcelona is hands down my most cherished city, and I would love to go back.

Costa Rica and Spain are two memorable places that I was blessed to explore. More importantly, they will always be dear to me because they were where I found myself. These two countries are where I discovered my passions, my patience and my strengths. They gave me the drive to continue travelling. You too can find your own Spain or Costa Rica.

A few years later, I took another trip, which was completely unique. I had the opportunity to visit my friend Natalie's parents' country. I travelled to Belgrade, Serbia to learn about my friend's culture, while at the same time seeing other nearby places such as Istanbul, Prague, and Dresden. These amazing cities were places that I would never have been to explore if I had not learned who I was as a person, and had not changed my attitude to enjoy every moment of my new life.

I understand that not everyone is in the position to travel or has the financial means to spend on elaborate vacations. I am aware that travelling is a luxury, and that it's hard to find time and money for it. And remember you do not have to travel far; just find your own nirvanas. My best suggestion is to look at your finances and perhaps meet with a financial planner to see if a trip is feasible. It never hurts to learn and discover what possibilities are out there.

Planning

That is the first thing I did when I was looking into travelling to Spain. I know that I am not the best at saving money. I am a professional spender. Let's just say that I have a bad habit of shopping, shopping, and shopping. Because I enjoy travelling, I decided to make some changes for myself and took the initiative to see a financial advisor. It was like going to therapy as I sat in the tiny office and spilled my story. I told her about my personal situation and about my goal to see Spain. She was patient and understanding. She agreed with me that a trip tends to cure stress of any kind. As we examined all of my options and ways for me to save money, I began to feel as though I had a plan. I was taking control of my situation and creating a goal for myself. Taking control of my desires made me feel as though I was redefining my life and myself.

In my bedroom, I have a GOAL jar. It is a simple old Mason jar with a sticker or word on it of my financial goal. I started keeping the jar many years ago. My jar sits on my bedside table so it is constantly within my sight. I collect only loonies and toonies in my jar. Once it is full, I roll up the coins and count my savings. Then every $500, I deposit my money into my savings account. I never spend my coins. I save them for my jar. In one year, I often collect almost $2000 and treat myself to a trip. This is one tactic to save money for a much-needed trip.

Even if a trip is completely out of the question for you in the next year, it is always something that you can plan for in the future. It boils down to creating goals, ambitions, dreams and desires that you want to see become a reality. I believe it is crucial for everyone to have a goal or a dream that they would like to see come true. Our passions drive us to success. If we have something we want badly enough, it will inevitably come true. I am not saying that your trip has to be to a foreign country or a tropical rainforest. I think even if you can get away to a new place in your backyard, you are still travelling. You are removing yourself from your current location and allowing new opportunities and experiences to enter your life. There are always nearby cities and places around you that are awaiting discovery. I would often spend weekends exploring cities that were close by. Venturing outside my familiar territory, even for a day or two, allowed me to forget my pain and feel free and independent.

I live in Mississauga, Ontario and would enjoy many weekends to nearby Stratford, or the Harbourfront in Toronto, Niagara-on-the-Lake, Muskoka, and Port Credit (only 20 minutes from my house) to escape my home area and build new memories for myself. Instead of sitting on my couch feeling sad and wallowing in self pity, I allowed myself to sit on the grass in Port Credit and snack on fruit while listening to music and discovering new restaurants in the area. I people watched and biked along the Harbourfront Centre in Toronto as I sipped hot chocolate and journalled by the water. One Saturday, I treated myself to a day trip to Niagara-on-the-Lake to walk the downtown area and browse through the boutiques offering samples of local wine and cheese. Having these little getaways allowed me to be proactive with my thoughts, feelings, and life experiences. These getaways were stepping stones to my healing and to creating a schedule of being active and training my brain to focus on positive thoughts.

I want to be clear and mention I am not anticipating if you go on a trip that all your pain, sorrow, and hurt will magically disappear; however, I do believe it will give you the lift you might need to heal. Nothing ventured, nothing gained! It is important to put your positive thoughts and realistic expectations on what it is exactly you want to gain from a trip. Travelling is an adventure. You are removing yourself from your present world and opening yourself to the unknown.

Travelling was exactly what I needed to help me heal, and appreciate and love myself. It forced me to be so grateful for each moment which made me realize that there was so much life out there to explore. I had my epiphany within those 10 days with Irina in Spain. My pain was disappearing and being replaced with happiness, dreams, aspirations, and realizing that I was better off in my new life. I was slowly becoming happy while being alone. I was becoming happy on my own. I was excited to see where my new life was going. I was happy being ME!

Recap:

- Look up places that intrigue you such as a museum or a famous restaurant or gallery in a city that you would like to visit. Spend a few minutes researching an area of interest and treat yourself to a day to explore and be adventurous. Adventure is within you; it is not in the place! Look within yourself and find your adventure. It is just around the corner.
- Write down places that you would love to discover and potential travelling buddies with whom to explore. Talking to friends who are interested in travelling gets the wheels in motion. It is helpful sharing travelling ideas and stories with others to create a plan and make it become a reality. It keeps the plan of a trip alive and keeps you focused on taking micro-steps to making it come true.
- Begin conversations with people about places that they have visited and openly listen to their stories. I always find that my best conversations with strangers or people I don't know extremely well revolve around travelling stories and their experiences. Hearing others talk about travelling might spark a destination you would love to explore.
- Take a look at your financial situation and areas in which you spend where you can begin saving and making cutbacks. Find ways to make money by having a garage sale, selling unwanted items and parting with jewelry or furniture that you don't need any more to begin saving your money for travel.

- Create your GOAL jar! Put it in a place where you can see it every day and it will become your constant reminder of what you are wanting in the future. In one year I saved almost $2000 in change and treated myself to a trip to Europe.
- Meet with a financial advisor at your bank and talk about your options in how to save extra money or allow the bank to take money directly out of your pay and put it into a separate account. This will prevent you from being tempted to spend it on other activities.

Chapter 8

Dating

"Dating has taught me what I want and don't want, who I am, and who I want to be."

-Jennifer Love Hewitt

I never anticipated writing a chapter on dating. That's because I never thought that I would have the strength to date. I am not recommending you date to move on in your healing necessarily, but I did find there were many positives to dating, that is, when you feel that you're finally comfortable with the idea.

Make sure before you get back into the dating scene that you have a sense of why you're doing it. You must be conscious of your expectations. I was not dating again to find my next soul mate. I simply needed to boost my confidence and build connections with interesting people. For me, dating was a way to learn about myself and be with people who enjoyed meeting and conversing over coffee. Some of the most interesting men that I met and lessons I learned occurred after I had met them. Not to mention, I built friendships with men and women along the way and cherished every new thing I learned whether it was big or small.

Before I got married, I dated and met many great men. I was a boy-crazy kind of gal who enjoyed wearing makeup, sporting the latest trends, and participating in social events where I might just meet "the one." When I moved to Toronto, I signed on to almost anything that would allow me to meet men. I tried speed dating, blind dates, and online dating. I would meet guys at parties, single functions, bars and clubs, and friends would hook me up with friends and family. While dating a guy, we usually communicated by phone. At the time, if I wanted to get to know someone or make arrangements for a dinner date, then it usually involved a phone call. When I met my ex-husband, people were still learning how to text. Then after my marriage dissolved, I had been out of the "dating" scene for several years. Times had changed and so had the dynamics of dating. Big time! Men and women acted differently with each other as the types of communication evolved. Everything that I had once understood as "dating" had drastically changed.

A few months after my separation, dancing became a must for me. As mentioned earlier, I needed to be around my girlfriends and music. Otherwise, I felt too alone with my thoughts. Talking to people and bonding with my girlfriends energized me and lifted my spirits. I decided to involve myself into social settings, even though, I felt insecure and unattractive after my failed marriage. I was honest with myself about not being interested in having a serious relationship, but I still wanted to believe there was hope I would find the 'right one.'

Ben

As mentioned earlier, I needed to be around my girlfriends and music. I simply enjoyed talking to people and bonding with my girlfriends. Since I was putting myself out into the social scene, I began meeting men who showed interest in taking me out for dinner and movies. Months into my separation, I met a young, Italian guy named Ben, who impressed me with flowers and chocolates at my door weekly. He and I often spent a lot of time together going to the movies and dining out at exciting restaurants. I immediately got swept up in the romance of spending time with a guy who was ten years younger than me and focusing my time and energy on reading his texts and listening to his laugh on the phone every night. Deep down, I knew that he and I were not going to become serious. He was aware of my situation. Even though it ended just as quickly as it began, he helped me realize many things about myself in a brief moment of time. On a superficial level, he introduced me to many fantastic restaurants in Toronto that are now some of my favourite places to dine. He made me feel beautiful and appreciate simple things like cups of coffee. I engaged in many inspiring discussions with him that showed me that I had much to offer and share in conversations. Most importantly, I believe his real purpose was to help me understand that I was capable of trusting. I did develop short term feelings for him and my energy and dedication quickly turned from my ex-husband towards Ben. I was trusting again. I was willing to take a chance and get to know someone. I learned that I was kind, patient, understanding, and forgiving and was not angry or wary with men. My anger and pain towards my ex was not affecting my outlook. I realized that during my dating journey, I was not in a negative place or position to hurt anyone. I remained true to who I was inside. I knew in my heart that I was going to be able to trust and believe in people. Even though Ben and I did not become a long term, romantic couple, he introduced me to many different places, made me laugh and taught me how to look at life differently. Ben pushed my limits and introduced me to the Auto Show, trendy restaurants, art galleries, and Twitter, and inspired me to have faith in my paintings.

Calvin

I met Calvin one night while out dancing. His charming demeanour and handsome good looks literally swept me off my feet. After that first encounter, he called to arrange a date with me. We had many things in common and enjoyed having intellectual conversations over bottles of foreign reds and Italian dishes. He opened my eyes to his culture, language, authors, and music. I cherished our closeness in restaurants while we watched funny videos on YouTube. He introduced me to his friends, treated me like a lady, and always had me laughing at his riddles and silly jokes. I thought I had died and gone to heaven. I found myself quickly falling for him and finding myself daydreaming about him.

The night before my trip to Europe, he called me on the phone and told me that he was not ready to be involved in a relationship. I actually got the "it's not you, it's me," line. Immediately following, I received the line," Do you want to be friends?" I felt like a high school girl being dumped on prom night. I was speechless. What happened? What had I done? Why had I not seen this coming?

On the flight to Serbia, I could not stop feeling hurt and empty inside. It brought to the surface a pain I hadn't felt since my ex-husband left. When I arrived in Belgrade, I told Natalie everything. She was extremely supportive and told me she would help me forget Calvin and that I would love my long-awaited trip. I knew that I would be fine in a couple of days once I was in a new place with my loving, nurturing friend.

I decided to look for the positive lessons that my experience with Calvin was teaching me. I learned that I had not lost anything, but instead gained something very powerful. Calvin taught me what it felt like to be treated like a classy lady, and how important laughter is to me in a relationship. He reminded me to enjoy the simple things and to find the beauty in romance once more. I realized the qualities that I saw in Calvin were qualities I wanted in a partner, and that they were things I was not willing to compromise on. He taught me that I do deserve to be treated like a lady, and that I have many wonderful qualities to offer someone. I ran into Calvin about six months later out one night and spoke to him with a non-confrontational and sincere attitude. When I saw his handsome face, I smiled instantly. I had wonderful memories with Calvin and I know deep down we will always laugh together whenever our paths cross.

Sam

I met Sam when I was out with my girlfriends. We exchanged phone numbers and texted right away. We met for dessert one night at Demetres. At the time, he had absolutely no idea that I was 12 years older than he was. I was honest about my age, but that did not seem to faze him. We continued texting, going to see movies, and meeting up for dinners or coffee. He heeded my restaurant and movie recommendations and would often send me messages that he had eaten at a pizza parlour I suggested, or had watched a film I loved. Months passed and it became clear to both of us that a serious relationship was not on the horizon.

After meeting one night at Starbucks, we agreed to be friends. Sam expressed to me that he admired my positive and optimistic attitude, and he admired my fortitude in the face of cancer. He was kind, and sincere, and he valued my thoughts and even liked my rants. For a few months, we took pleasure in each other's conversations, yet as the months past, I saw less and less of him.

Months later, I received an anonymous email from a woman saying that she had heard about me from someone but did not feel comfortable telling me who it was. I was unsure if I wanted to reply, yet something told me that she was genuine and honest. After several emails back and forth, I later found out that she knew Sam, and that he had spoken very highly about me. Tamara was a kind woman and a fan of my blog. I agreed to meet her for coffee and the beginning of a new friendship was developing. Meeting Sam had given me the gift of a new friend in Tamara. She is a friend who values me just the way I am and inspires me to see the good in people, to give, and to always be genuine. We both believe it is important to keep positive people in our lives.

Hadi

Hadi and I instantly clicked and decided for our first date to meet at a restaurant for a glass of wine. Once again, a committed relationship never grew with Hadi, but what I do remember most about him was that he believed in me. He listened attentively to my visions about publishing my book and wanting to be a part of Cook for the Cure. I remember on our first date, Hadi wanted to sponsor me and asked how he could be involved. At the time, I figured he was just trying to impress me; however, there was something in his eyes that made me think he was honest. Together we talked about our dreams and goals, and we both inspired each other with deep conversations about how to make them a reality.

Hadi admired my determination and made me feel confident and unique. At the same time, he taught me to follow my dreams and to have faith in myself. Today Hadi and I no longer keep in touch, but we ended on good terms, and he is a positive memory in my mind of somebody who gave me the courage to complete my book and believe in something inside of me, even when I had doubts of my own.

At Chapters Indigo I found a wealth of books published on dating such as Men Are From Mars Women Are From Venus, On Your Own Again, and Modern Dating to name but a few. All of these titles and many more offer helpful tips on dating dos and don'ts. While browsing through these books, I learned tips ranging from what colours to wear on a date to suggesting time frames on when it is appropriate to return calls or text back. Some suggested not talking too much on a date while other books suggested talking as much as you could to show your confidence. Much of the dating wisdom in these books had been around for years, while other information was new and relevant.

These books offer many different dating tactics to choose from, so they are not made for everyone. I would suggest going to the bookstore and selecting one that feels right for you. If you try to implement all the dating rules in these books, it could be too overwhelming and the "dater" could sabotage the date and possibilities for happiness altogether. Keep an open mind while reading a book about dating. Select rules that bring comfort to you and follow your own beliefs and morals. Most important "be yourself" as this is the best rule to follow, and there is also nothing wrong with bringing new ideas to the table.

Above all, remember that dating is fun, positive, and a bit of a learning curve. The rules and players in this game are constantly evolving and adapting. People will always bring their own experiences and knowledge into dating. As I've demonstrated, whether short term or long term, you can build amazing connections with people you meet. Everyone offers a new perspective, or a story to share. Everyone is different and looking for something different. As long as you are true to yourself and are confident about what it is you are looking for, then things will always work out for the best. This epiphany surrounding dating did not strike me on the first couple of dates.

No! No! No! I became more experienced and stronger the more I dated. I endured my fair share of crying and heartache. I have had many bad dates and met some interesting men to say the least. I have been stood up, left at restaurants for hours waiting, not received expected phone calls and had the line, "I am not ready for a commitment" shoved in my face on numerous occasions. Many times, I wanted to give up and burrow my head into my pillow. I often blamed myself; however, I never gave up. Giving up was not a concept I knew or practised any more.

It took me a long time to appreciate and perceive dating as experiences, knowledge, lessons, and connections. I may not have met the "right" guy for me, but I was enjoying the dating journey and relishing times when I shared my stories with my girlfriends. I was learning about the world around me and about the interesting people living in it. Finding the positive in each moment is something I have made a point of consistently crafting for myself. Many of my friends kept telling me to take it easy or to stop dating altogether. This was good and sincere advice as I knew my friends wanted the best for me, and a part of me knew they were right. I could not stop though because I knew that heartbreaks and failed dating were making me stronger and teaching me more about myself. I do not regret one date that I went on or one to whom I gave a chance. I see the positive. That is who I am. Dating was an experience that opened my eyes to the type of man I did want. It showed me the values and characteristics that were important to me in a partner. I began to understand and accept traits that were attractive to me, and how those traits made me feel as a human.

Recap: Date Only When You're Ready

- Remember you are dating to meet people and build connections NOT looking for another marriage partner.
- Look into dating sites, speed dating, single events, parties, and most importantly put yourself out there. You will never meet people sitting on your couch. People are out there! So find your smile and start mingling.
- Be open and be yourself.

- Ask your friends to help you create a dating profile. Grab a coffee and have your friends describe you the way they truly see you. We can be our own worst critics.
- Say, YES YES YES to every invitation. You never know who you might meet.
- Remember to show up on time, dress classy, be talkative and a good listener, be yourself and have FUN!

Chapter 9

Say Yes

"Always say 'yes' to the present moment... Surrender to what is. Say 'yes' to life - and see how life starts suddenly working for you rather than against you."

-Eckhart Tolle

Say Yes!

This chapter represents the most important advice about taking your life back and moving on to discovering what you are meant to do. I sympathize and empathize with your pain. Separation is never easy whether it is amicable or not. Maybe your marriage is ending, and you feel lost and uncertain about where you are headed. An unusual feeling sinks in, and you are consumed with many conflicting emotions that don't make sense. I'm going to introduce you to a little exercise that has helped me. Try to refocus your thoughts on positive things, people and words, starting with the word, YES. This is the word that is going to be the most powerful word in your vocabulary and the word with the most integrity.

First, tell yourself that "YES, I am going to heal." "YES, I am strong and will move on." "YES, I am good person and deserve the best." Change the way your mind thinks and it will change everything you feel too. Once you develop a routine of using this word for yourself and in your language, it will be time to put it into practice.

Say YES to everything (or as much as you possibly can). You will be invited to events by friends and asked to do things with your family. Opportunities to participate in different activities will begin to present themselves to you. This is the time; you are putting the word YES into action.

Becoming involved in different activities offers opportunities for you to learn, contribute and build connections. Keeping yourself busy and involved gives you a sense of accomplishment and acceptance. Saying NO to offers, events, or opportunities will only close doors to the world and all it has to offer. Saying NO too many times will consume you and your spirit. Friends and family might stop asking you altogether to participate in events. Say YES to a variety of different things and the universe will give you a world of amazing opportunities.

Some of my most memorable YES moments that occurred during my separation opened incredible doors for me that changed the course of my life and expanded my horizons.

Due to the many YESES in my life, I have started a blog, raised money for cancer research, attended a Madonna concert, gone to the Queen's Plate horse race, attended many food events, met Canadian celebrity chefs, travelled, won second place in a Purdy's chocolate contest, got a tattoo, started entering my photos in competitions, modelled for Leigh and Harlow clothing store, and of course, travelled.

Saying YES to one thing led me to say YES to other things.

One day, I received a call from Amy who invited me to model some clothing for a Toronto clothing store. Of course, without hesitation, I said, you guessed it, YES. I had a super time that day with Amy. I met her friend and photographer Jeff Turner who took amazing photographs of me on his motorcycle, by the waters in Port Credit, and against a wall wearing the latest trends. I felt alive and confident. I later saw my face on Leigh and Harlow's webpage and fell in love with their clothing. As months passed, Jeff Turner contacted me and asked me if I wanted to be involved in his upcoming event called The Me Project. The Me Project is an artist photography exhibit featuring many women who have survived or are battling cancer. Of course, without hesitation, I said YES. I met Jeff one sunny Monday afternoon in August, and he found a secluded area in natural setting to photograph me. The shots were tasteful and artistic. I felt a part of something much bigger and was proud of myself for getting involved in a cause that is dear to me.

Another example of saying YES is this book's publication. Don't get me wrong. Yes, the topic of this book was created out of a terrible incident in my life; however, the work and the connections to have it completed are only an amazing result of saying YES. As I have mentioned, since I can remember, I have wanted to publish a book. It was not until my separation and driving desire to share my experiences with others that I knew what that book that would be. Saying YES to coming to Starbucks once a week for several months to focus on my writing was a huge contributing factor to this book's completion.

Saying YES to one positive thing snowballed into something more powerful than I could ever imagine. During these past two years after my separation, I have worked hard at saying YES and made making a conscious effort to meet new people and gain as much knowledge as possible.

Another example of how my YES theory made my life better was when I attended a writing course. I drove 45 minutes out of my way after work to learn about taking criticism and employing some powerful writing tips. I attended many workshops all over Toronto on how to publish a novel and arranged meeting authors in the area. I also spent time researching books at the library about the industry. As often as possible, I was also constantly approaching authors and sharing with them my desire to publish a book. I joined an on-line writers group and entered writing contests to keep myself involved in my writing.

By saying yes you are removing yourself from your present world and opening yourself to the unknown.

I basically said YES to trying everything related to writing and seized any opportunity that came my way. At the end of the day, the success of my book being published was ultimately up to me and not anyone else.

Saying YES will always open a door or two and will keep you motivated, I promise you. I was able to publish a book because I believed in saying YES.

Of course, the biggest YES that brought incredible riches into my life was saying YES to fighting cancer with healthy food. I said YES to a naturopath, a juicer, cooking, a natural lifestyle and healing books, alternative medicines, positive thinking, advice and support from friends and family, attending every doctor's appointment, going to the gym weekly, and focusing on my dream to climb the Eiffel Tower on my fifth year. During my first year of treatment, I had made up my mind to climb this historical monument after reaching my five-year remission mark. That summer after receiving my good news of remaining in remission, I planned a trip to travel through Bosnia, Croatia, Montenegro, and finally Paris. My excitement peaked the day I arrived in Paris. I remember seeing the Eiffel Tower for the first time and becoming captured by its stunning beauty and height above the rooftops and cathedral spires. I had never seen anything so breathtaking. I was in love with the city and eager for my climb. The day I ascended to the top of the tower, the sun beamed in a cloudless sky. When I reached the top, I looked down on the city of Paris and felt a sense of peace overwhelm me. I felt a large weight lift from my body and a lightness to my limbs. I had accomplished one of my dreams and was now at the top of the Eiffel Tower. The top of the world. My YES theory brought me to that moment.

Another YES moment that brought wonderful opportunity into my life occurred when I received an email from Rethink, a Canadian charity that supports and brings awareness to women diagnosed with breast cancer. Rethink invited me to attend the Queen's Plate at Woodbine Racetrack in Toronto. I remember opening the invitation and thinking that it seemed too good to be true. I would be in the VIP tent where complimentary food and drinks would be offered. It would be a chance to dress up and wear a unique hat and mingle with people while supporting awareness for my cause. It was an opportunity of a lifetime. I couldn't believe I was being invited to such an extravagant event. The only drawback was that I was only offered one ticket. I was not sure I could attend an event solo and find the courage for a whole afternoon to meet people on my own. I ponder the thought for many days and then remembered my say YES motto. This was yet another opportunity for me to stand up and be counted, especially for something I wholeheartedly believed in. I emailed the coordinator back and thanked her graciously and then began my hunt for a big hat that would stand out.

It was a sunny Sunday afternoon. The Woodbine Racetrack was bustling with people and vendors standing under large white tents. I walked towards the entrance, my heart racing and adrenaline rushing through my veins. I entered a beautiful pink decorated tent, my assigned tent for the afternoon. There was an open bar, appetizers, a table decorated with candy and a photo booth. I gracefully sat on a leather couch in the sun and gazed at the crowds while snacking on treats in my flouncy blue hat.

As the day progressed, I met some interesting people and was introduced to my newest food obsession, Pad Thai fries. It was the greatest thing I had ever tasted. I was so grateful for the complimentary food that was donated to this cause that I decided to find the chef or provider and thank him personally. There was a large red food truck behind the tent that said "Fidel Gastro." I sauntered over and introduced myself to the owner, a young, magnanimous guy named Matt Basile. After thanking him for supporting the cause and telling him how much I loved Pad Thai fries, he mentioned that he owned a restaurant called Lisa Marie and invited me to check it out for dinner.

As the months passed, I not only visited his restaurant often, but also tracked his truck around town, tracked him on Twitter, won a copy of his cookbook, celebrated Halloween and New Year's Eve at Lisa Marie and developed a friendship with Matt. I enjoyed supporting his cookbook by taking pictures of it everywhere I went and posting it over different forms of social media.

Matt was extremely down to earth, full of energy, inspiring, and an overall kind person, so I wanted to show my support to him anyway I could. One day, Matt even suggested I be a part of the audience in an upcoming episode for the television show, "You Gotta Eat Here." His restaurant would be featured on the show. Are you kidding me? What an honour. YES! YES! YES! Being part of the show's taping was exciting and rewarding. I got to meet the host, John Catucci, eat a ton of tasty food, and once again, meet interesting people.

By saying YES to one simple event, life led me on many new adventures. I can proudly say that I attended a major event by myself made the most of it and overcame my fear. I fell in love with Pad Thai fries and built a friendship with one of Toronto's most successful and talented chefs and restaurant owners, Matt Basile. I was asked to be a guest on a Canadian television series and was interviewed about the food I tasted by host John Catucci. This day was an opportunity for me, and a memory that I was excited to share. I felt honoured to be part of this experience with Matt, and I built a friendship with another Canadian hero of mine, whom I admire as an entrepreneur and as a person.

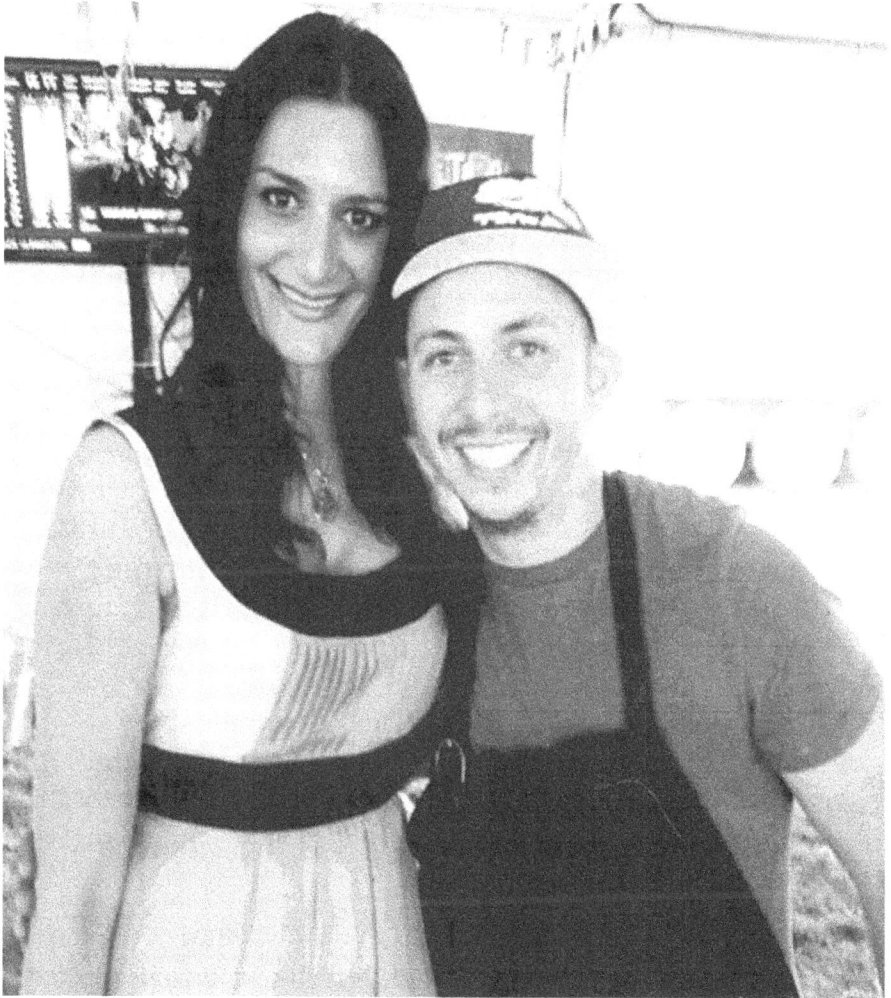

Matt Basile

Mind you, saying Yes, may involve you confronting your fears.

I know facing the unknown is not easy. Everyone has different levels of strengths and confidence when engaging in unfamiliar activities. Fears hold us back from exploring, self discovery, and experiences. Some of us have many fears, while others have few. Some of us can control our fears and cope with them daily, while others are constantly wanting to overcome them. Some of us have fears that are new, while others have fears that have remained in their lives for a long time. I also want to emphasize that having fears is natural and necessary. It is part of being human. We need them. Fears keep us safe and protect us from danger. They teach us how to rationalize and how to understand our intuition. Fear inspires us to live by challenging us to create success and to grow. Fear is contagious. We share stories about our accomplishments that might enlighten others to create their own stories. Perhaps, sharing my story about facing my fear of heights and zip lining in Costa Rica might inspire you to do the same.

Walking away from a bad relationship, standing up to your boss, quitting your job, moving to a new city, or de-cluttering your home from things that might have sentimental value are all things involve facing your fears and helping you move on. They require a personal change or a personal risk. Moving on from a separation and forcing yourself to challenge and confront your fears demonstrates your strength. Once you confront your fears and challenge yourself, you begin to feel liberated. You will have started the journey of opening doors to other new and exciting opportunities.

When I was going through depression and separation anxiety, I recall my friend Stephanie telling me to visualize a swimming pool.

Many people are in the pool coasting along in the middle of the water and enjoying a comfortable swim with no fear of drowning or sinking," she said. "Hitting rock bottom is sinking to the bottom of the pool and making the choice to land on your feet using your energy to push yourself back up to the top of the water to breathe. If you choose too, you only have up to go. You have the strength and the drive to take control of your decision and force yourself to push yourself to better limits."

Creating this book has allowed me to take my personal tragedy and turn it into a positive experience by helping me to accomplish my goals. I said "YES" to change, to facing my fears, and to learning about my inner strength.

Recap

- SAY YES TODAY
- AND EVERYDAY!

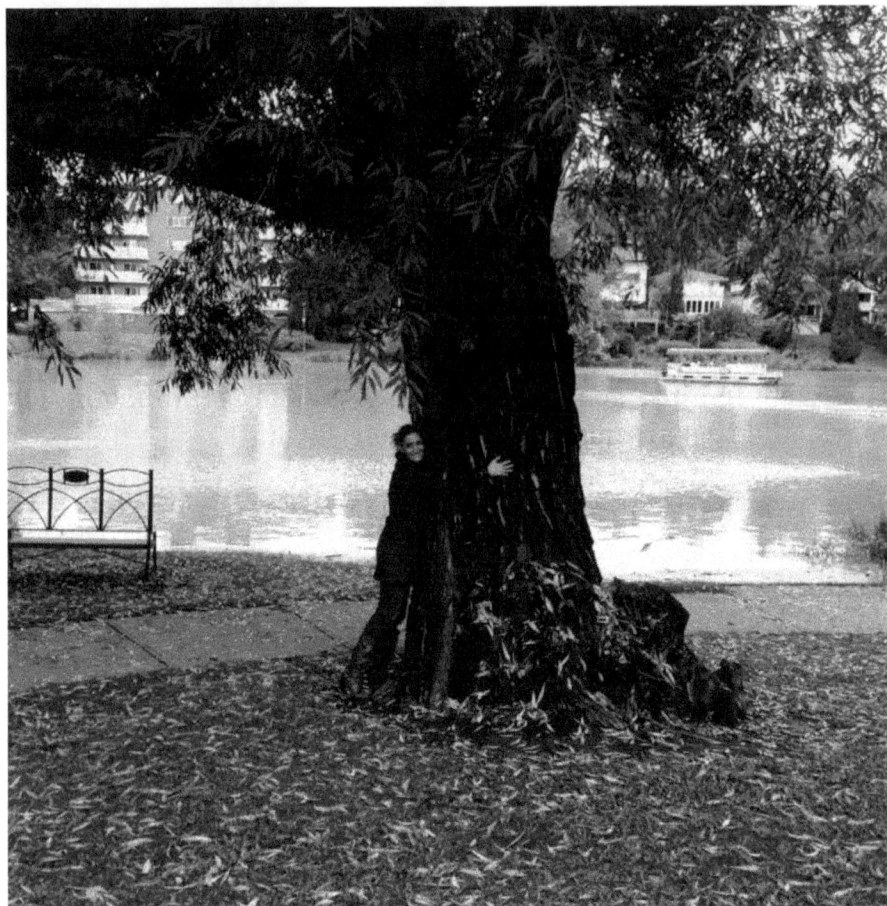

Getting back into nature

Conclusion: Final Thoughts

"Do not pray for an easy life, pray for the strength to endure a difficult one."

-Bruce Lee

With this book, I set out to inspire and help you cope with the pains and heartache of dealing with a broken heart. I wish to offer suggestions and strategies that I used myself to help me move on and find a better, more positive life. I know that not everything I have suggested will suit everyone or fit every situation. My intent is simply to share my story honestly and openly, in hopes that you, the reader, will take away some wisdom, and feel hopeful that you are closer to being where you want to be in your life.

Perhaps you will come upon an idea in these pages that triggers an inspiration and helps you on your journey to recovery. Perhaps this book has been sitting on your desk or your coffee table for a while before you decide to pick it up. Either way, my intent in writing and sharing my story with you is truly to help and inspire.

In the end, writing this book was therapeutic and helped me to heal and build my confidence on my path to recovery. Rereading my work three years later reminded me of all of my accomplishments, strengths, talents, and of all the riches that are mine. I am a happy, confident, strong, passionate, and inspiring woman who has a story to tell.

Three years ago, I would have never imagined being in my present position in my life. I would not have met Vikram Vij or met one of my favourite Canadian chefs, Michael Smith. I would have not written this book, travelled to amazing places, bonded with inspirational people, cooked exotic meals, painted pictures, golfed, obtained a makeup certificate, or felt the powers of gratitude if I had not endured my painful separation. My point is simple. Good things will happen. Trust me. You will see why you are given challenges and pain. In time, if you are patient, you will find your own inner strength and become stronger than you thought possible. Though I am offering you hope to make it through difficult times, you have the power to find your strength to create your own future.

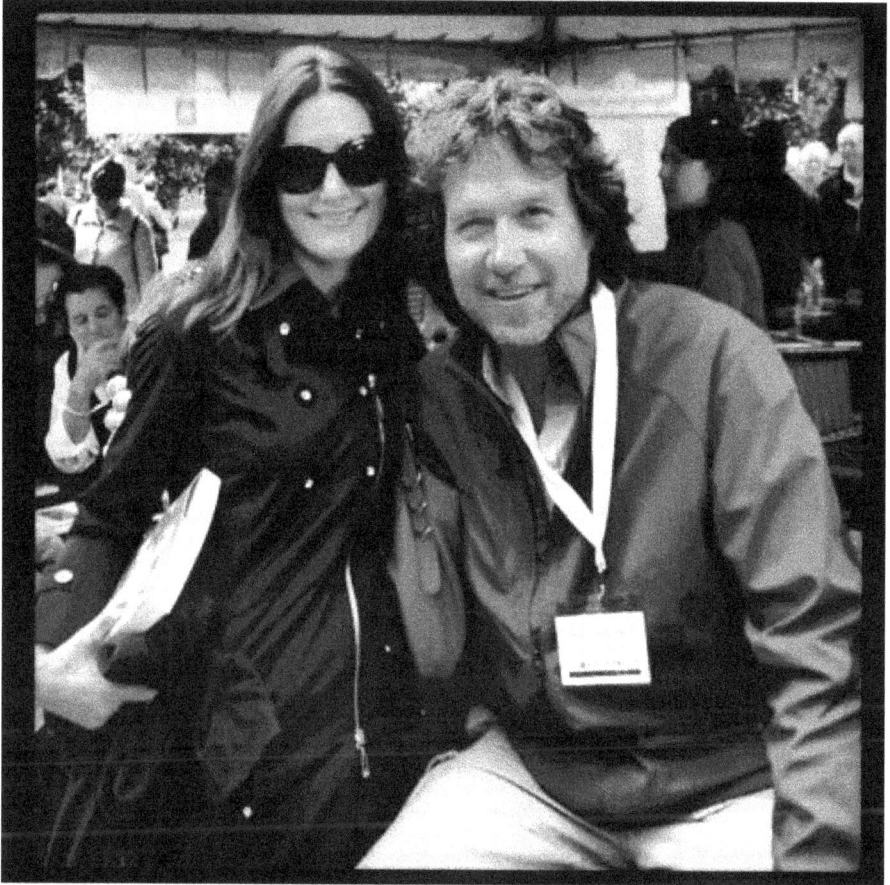

Michael Smith and I

I am appreciative for the amazing experiences and people that I have met on my journey. I have made the conscious decision to look at things in a positive light and to feel grateful for all that I have in my life. Even though my heart was broken and life did not seem fair, I knew that I had to keep moving on, even if my steps were tiny. We are all in control of our own decisions and the way we deal and cope with life's mysteries.

I titled my book Wide Awake because it was not until I had undergone the pain and loss that I became "wide awake" to my situation and could see clearly why things had unfolded the way they had. My eyes were shut during the process, and for a short time, I could only see the negative and what I perceived as the impossible. I never imagined the amazing opportunities that awaited me. Things happen for a reason. Yet, I had to search for them. I had a choice to see things differently, and I made that choice. I had the power to open my eyes and see what I wanted to see. My eyes were not shut anymore. They were wide awake and what I chose to see finally were endless possibilities and a new beginning.

A final thought to end this book: A shout out to all who are experiencing a broken heart and have lost hope. Please believe that you will heal eventually and that wonderful adventures and connections await you; however, your fate and happiness lie within your hands. It is time for you to take back your life and discover all that awaits. For life is a journey, not a destination. Become the creator of your adventures. Take charge of your decisions and make the necessary changes.

Reading this book is a baby step to healing and being open to strategies that will help you. I would strongly encourage you to please email me or message me on Facebook or Twitter to share what has helped you begin on your healing journey. We all have a story to tell. I have shared my story with you. What is yours?

Be your own inspiration!

mody365@hotmail.com

@SModyBIA

Epilogue

It has been several years now since my separation began and my divorce was finalized. As I look back at that time in my life, I have learned many things about myself and improved immensely my ways of thinking. Life will always throw curve balls at us. It is a part of what "living" is all about. At the same time, we are also given the choice and strength to overcome any situation and to move on with our lives. In simpler terms, when life gives you lemons, make lemonade. Gratitude has become a part of how I choose to live my life and where I find my greatest strength. I am grateful for the places I have travelled to and for those I will continue to discover. I am grateful for the people who I have met and for the ones still to meet. I am grateful each day for my health and for all the energy and stability it provides me. I am grateful for the experiences I have in memory and the ones on my Bucket List. Every day I wake up, I am happy for my family and friends that have continually provided me with love and support, and for love I know they will gladly give me in the years to come. My life has taken a turn for the best and it is simply a choice that I make for myself; a choice that continues to provide me with wondrous possibilities. I never imagined that my life could begin all over again when many things seemed to be ending and falling apart all around me. To this day, I still actively volunteer, attend concerts, conferences and local events, travel, cook, exercise, dance, write, blog, and spend time with family and friends. I seize opportunities as they come. I choose to live in the present and leave my past behind.

I am wide awake.

Original Journal Entries

Feb 2	I am grateful for my talents.
Feb 1	I am grateful for my legs.
Jan 31	I am grateful for my education.
Jan 30	I am grateful for my love of animals.
Jan 29	I am grateful for my hair. oops!
Jan 28	I am grateful for loving tea.
Jan 27	I am grateful for my experiences.
Jan 26	I am grateful for my genetics.
Jan 25	I am grateful for my classroom.
Jan 24	I am grateful for my laugh.
Jan 23	I am grateful for my kind ♡
Jan 22	I am grateful for my benefits.
Jan 21	I am grateful for my garden.
Jan 20	I am grateful for my home.
Jan 19	I am grateful for my eyesight.
Jan 18	I am grateful for my hair
Jan 17	I am grateful for my car.
Jan 16	I am grateful for education
Jan 15	I am grateful for my travels
Jan 14	I am grateful for my cats.
Jan 13	I am grateful for my career.
Jan 12	I am grateful for my health.
Jan 11	I am grateful for my friends.
Jan 10th	I am grateful for my family

Feb 26	I am grateful for vegetables.
Feb 25	I am grateful for fruit.
Feb 24	I am grateful for nature.
Feb 23	I am grateful for outgoing personality.
Feb 22	I am grateful for my summer off
Feb 21	I am grateful for my teeth.
Feb 20	I am grateful for Family Day!
Feb 19	I am grateful for Irina
Feb 18	I am grateful for my voice
Feb 17	I am grateful for my strength.
Feb 16	I am grateful for meeting Benjamin
Feb 15	I am grateful for movies.
Feb 14	I am grateful for friends.
Feb 13	I am grateful for knowing how to swim.
Feb 12	I am grateful for being able to read.
Feb 11	I am grateful for my kind heart
Feb 10	I am grateful for chocolate.
Feb 9	I am grateful for my country.
Feb 8	I am grateful for my love of art.
Feb 7	I am grateful for my strength.
Feb 6	I am grateful for my sister.
Feb 5	I am grateful for hair. (again)
Feb 4	I am grateful for my soul.
Feb 3	I am grateful for my smile.

March 21	I am grateful for supportive neighbours.
March 20	I am grateful for meeting Liz at an Irish Bar.
March 19	I am grateful for fresh air.
March 18	I am grateful for being literate.
March 17	I am grateful for having good morals.
March 16	I am grateful for Benjamin's laugh.
March 15	I am grateful for love of life.
March 14	I am grateful for my March Break.
March 13	I am grateful for my braces.
March 12	I am grateful for enjoying golf.
March 11	I am grateful for having no allergies.
March 10	I am grateful for my background.
March 9	I am grateful for my nose.
March 8	I am grateful for my positive outlook.
March 7	I am grateful for Janaki
March 6	I am grateful for photography talents.
March 5	I am grateful that I can swim.
March 4	I am grateful for Orillia
March 3	I am grateful for my cancer free body.
March 2	I am grateful for the amazing women I meet.
March 1	I am grateful for water.
Feb 29	I am grateful for my holidays.
Feb 28	I am grateful for hot days.
Feb 27	I am grateful for Jen Stolk.

April 15	I am grateful to have a pension.
April 14	I am grateful for my income.
April 13	I am grateful for good listeners.
April 12	I am grateful for my healthy heart.
April 11	I am grateful for my toes.
April 10	I am grateful for waterfalls.
April 9	I am grateful for tears.
April 8	I am grate for time.
April 7	I am grateful for Nilmini
April 6	I am grateful for love.
April 5	I am grateful for medicine
April 4	I am grateful for pancakes.
April 3	I am grateful for latin clubs.
April 2	I am grateful for trees.
April 1	I am grateful that most people like me ☺
March 30	I am grateful for having trust for others.
March 29	I am grateful for sunshine.
March 28	I am grateful for my positive childhood memories.
March 27	I am grateful for learning how to play the
March 26	I am grateful for being able to run.
March 25	I am grateful for yoga! ☺
March 24	I am grateful for Bonnie Ross.
March 23	I am grateful for my determination.
March 22	I am grateful for my health care.

May 9	I am grateful my dad's love.
May 8	I am grateful for cardinals.
May 7	I am grateful for my determination.
May 6	I am grateful for my voice.
May 5	I am grateful for bumblebees.
May 4	I am grateful for Janis.
May 3	I am grateful for raspberries.
May 2	I am grateful that I enjoy helping others.
May 1	I am grateful for my passion for life.
April 30	I am grateful for comedies.
April 29	I am grateful for grass.
April 28	I am grateful for meditation
April 27	I am grateful for Carol Morley.
April 26	I am grateful for my love of scrabble.
April 25	I am grateful my fathers hugs.
April 24	I am grateful for my mom's advice.
April 23	I am grateful for shampoo.
April 22	I am grateful for Earth day!
April 21	I am grateful for Zen tea.
April 20	I am grateful for the rain.
April 19	I am grateful for being treated like a lady
April 18	I am grateful for cell phones.
April 17	I am grateful for butterflies.
April 16	I am grateful for the flowers I received on my birthday.

May 31 I am grateful for sand.
May 30 I am grateful for pimple cream.
May 29 I am grateful for Tazo Ice Tea.
May 28 I am grateful for shampoo + conditioner
May 27 I am grateful for birds.
May 26 I am grateful for meeting Sony.
May 25 I am grateful for my dads unconditional love.
May 24 I am grateful for Matt Muhlond
May 23 I am grateful for people who hold the
May 22 I am grateful for long sleeps. door open.
May 21 I am grateful for clean water.
May 20 I am grateful for a cat's purr.
May 19 I am grateful for Tony at the water store
May 18 I am grateful for being able to swim.
May 17 I am grateful for being able to drive.
May 16 I am grateful for eggs benedict.
May 15 I am grateful for pretty jewlery.
May 14 I am grateful for charities.
May 13 I am grateful for my ability to golf.
May 12 I am grateful for people's kindness.
May 11 I am grateful for Paul Barao.
May 10 I am grateful for red wine.